Heart Disease

Heart Disease

Rob Myers, MD, FRCPC

KEY PORTER BOOKS

To my wife, Randi Cheryl, and my kids, Seth Noah Jarrett, Rachel Fawn, and Aaron Hunter Joseph—RM

National Library of Canada Cataloguing-in-Publication Data

Myers, Rob
    Heart disease / Rob Myers.

Includes bibliographical references and index.
ISBN 1-55263-268-7

1. Heart—Diseases—Popular works. I. Title.

RC682.M94 2004   616.1'2   C2003-905174-9

THE CANADA COUNCIL | LE CONSEIL DES ARTS
FOR THE ARTS | DU CANADA
SINCE 1957 | DEPUIS 1957

ONTARIO ARTS COUNCIL
CONSEIL DES ARTS DE L'ONTARIO

The publisher gratefully acknowledges the support of the Canada Council for the Arts and the Ontario Arts Council for its publishing program.

We acknowledge the financial support of the Government of Canada through the Book Publishing Industry Development Program (BPIDP) for our publishing activities.

We acknowledge the support of the Government of Ontario through the Ontario Media Development Corporation's Ontario Book Initiative.

Key Porter Books Limited
70 The Esplanade
Toronto, Ontario
Canada M5E 1R2

www.keyporter.com

Design: Peter Maher
Electronic formatting: Heidy Lawrance Associates

This book is not a substitute for medical diagnosis and you are advised to always consult your physician for specific information on personal health matters.

Printed and bound in Canada

04 05 06 07 08 09 6 5 4 3 2 1

Contents

Introduction

Everyone knows someone with heart disease, whether that someone is a parent or sibling, boss or neighbor, friend or acquaintance. Heart ailments are so common, it is nearly impossible to remain untouched. Cardiovascular disease, which includes heart attacks and strokes, is the leading cause of death in North America. It is responsible for 37 percent of all deaths, and is the most common cause of death for those over sixty-five. At all ages, death rates from heart disease are much greater in men than in women.

Despite the morbid tone of the above, there is reason to be optimistic. The past thirty years have shown a dramatic decline in mortality (death) rates from heart disease. Between 1975 and 1995 (the date of the last available statistics), the mortality rate within the first thirty days after a heart attack dropped 63 percent. In other words, although heart disease still strikes, we are now more likely to live with it than die from it.

Directly or indirectly, heart disease will affect everyone reading this book. How we deal with the problem is, in large part, a matter of education. Few of us spend enough time educating ourselves about common health problems. Ignorance may be bliss, but premature death is a more likely result. When it comes to health and disease, many people are mired in a lethal combination of fear and avoidance. This problem is compounded by the fact that sometimes physicians have trouble explaining medical concepts simply and clearly. If a famous writer like Stephen King wrote about heart ailments, more people would pay attention—although they still might end up too scared to do anything about them.

Too many books make cardiology—the branch of medicine related to heart problems—as interesting as the instruction booklet for your new dishwasher. But cardiology, like medicine in general, is easier to understand than most people realize. The desire to learn, to read and to implement change will increase your longevity and improve your quality of life. The weeks it may take to navigate through, and understand, medical jargon can easily translate into a happier and healthier life.

In this book, the medical terms you need are defined in the text, and many also appear in the glossary at the end of the book. Complex topics are explained in straightforward, everyday language. Drugs are identified by their generic names, but common brand names are listed in the drug table at the end.

I hope you will take the time to read and reread this book. I believe you will also find it a useful reference. The small amount of time and effort required can help you, and those close to you, on the road to a happier, healthier life.

R.M.

1. The Normal Heart

You cannot understand heart disease without first learning the words and phrases that physicians use to discuss it. Familiarity with the basic anatomy of the heart is a good starting point.

The heart is about the size of a softball, and it resides under the ribs of the left side of the chest. It's a muscle, but unlike the muscles of the rest of our body it works twenty-four hours a day without a break, and does not normally fatigue. This makes sense, as it must pump about forty to one hundred times a minute for the life of its owner. This may add up to over three billion beats for someone who lives past seventy years of age and has a typical average heart rate of about seventy beats per minute.

The heart's job is to deliver blood laden with oxygen and other nutrients to the body. It also accepts the oxygen-poor blood from the head and body and pumps it back to the lungs to pick up a fresh supply of oxygen. Blood is pumped away from the heart through thick-walled *arteries*, and returns to the heart through thin-walled *veins*.

Four chambers make up the heart: the *right atrium, right ventricle, left atrium* and *left ventricle*. There are also four valves—the *tricuspid, pulmonic, mitral* and *aortic*. The valves ensure that blood flows in only one direction. Blood arrives at the right atrium of the heart through veins from the head and body. It crosses the tricuspid valve into the right ventricle and is pumped across the pulmonic valve into the lungs to pick up oxygen. From the lungs it moves into the left atrium, crosses the mitral valve into the left ventricle and is pumped across the aortic valve, through the aorta (the main artery) and into lesser arteries to deliver this oxygen to the head and body.

Blood circulation of the heart and lungs

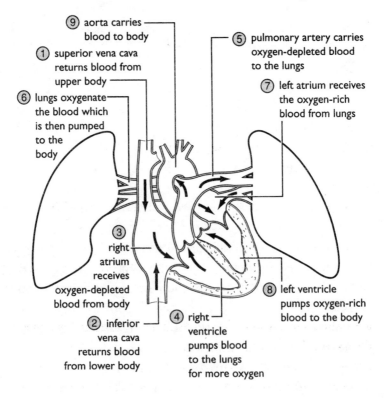

⑨ aorta carries blood to body

① superior vena cava returns blood from upper body

⑥ lungs oxygenate the blood which is then pumped to the body

⑤ pulmonary artery carries oxygen-depleted blood to the lungs

⑦ left atrium receives the oxygen-rich blood from lungs

③ right atrium receives oxygen-depleted blood from body

② inferior vena cava returns blood from lower body

④ right ventricle pumps blood to the lungs for more oxygen

⑧ left ventricle pumps oxygen-rich blood to the body

The coronary arteries

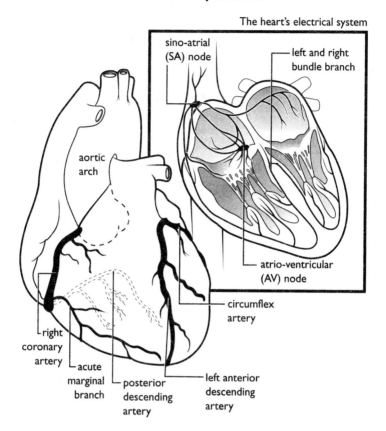

The heart's electrical system

The heart also has its own blood vessels, the *coronary arteries*. Just as water flows through branches of a tree to nourish the leaves, blood flows through the coronary arteries to feed the heart. The three main arteries are the *right coronary artery* (*RCA*), the *circumflex artery* (*CX*) and the *left anterior descending artery* (*LAD*). The important branches of the LAD are called *septals* and *diagonals*. The important branches of the circumflex are called *obtuse marginals*. The RCA has a *posterior descending* and *posterolateral* branch. One of the reasons it takes so long to complete medical school is the need to to memorize all these strange names.

The heart also has specialized electrical "wiring" that carries signals to the muscle, resulting in a heartbeat. An electrical impulse is initiated in the *sino-atrial* (*SA*) node. It passes through the atria to the *atrio-ventricular* (*AV*) node. This node separates the atria and ventricles electrically. From the AV node, the electrical impulse activates the left and right ventricles through branches called the left and right *bundle branch*.

With its rooms (chambers), doors (valves), plumbing (coronary arteries) and electrical system, the heart is rather like a house. Like a house—unfortunately—it sometimes has things go wrong.

2. Risk Factors for Heart Disease

D riving defensively at the speed limit lowers the odds that you will be involved in an accident, but it cannot negate the possibility. Similarly, with simple lifestyle changes that focus on smoking cessation, exercise and a balanced diet, the chances of a heart attack can be dramatically reduced, but they will never drop to zero.

Modifiable and Unmodifiable Risk Factors

The risk factors for heart disease are well known to most people. They are easily divided into those that can be changed and those that cannot. Sex cannot be changed; men are more likely to develop *coronary artery disease* (*CAD*) than women, and they do so at a younger age. In 1997, in the United States, men between the ages of twenty-nine and forty-four had 126,000 heart attacks, but women in the same age group had only 3,000 heart attacks.

Age is also an unalterable risk factor. The older we are, the greater the risk of most diseases, including heart disease.

Risk Factors

What we can't change	What we can change
sex	smoking
age	high blood pressure
family history	high cholesterol
	diabetes control
	significant obesity

Family history is another risk factor we can't change. But having a family member with heart disease is not an automatic death sentence. Family history is considered relevant only if a first-degree male relative (father or brother) has had a heart attack, *angioplasty* or bypass surgery before the age of fifty-five, and/or a first-degree female relative (mother or sister) has had the same before age sixty-five. (Angioplasties and bypass surgery are both used to treat heart disease.) Accordingly, a history of a heart attack in a second cousin twice removed is meaningless in terms of your risk, just as a great-great-grand-mother who died suddenly after being scared by a horse is irrelevant to your health.

High Blood Pressure (Hypertension)

The pressure exerted by blood flowing in the arteries is called blood pressure (BP). When the heart contracts, it propels blood into the aorta, the body's main artery. The arteries that supply our organs and other body parts branch off from the aorta like branches off a tree trunk. A number of factors can lead to higher-than-normal blood pressure, also called *hypertension*.

Blood-pressure problems plague almost one in five North Americans. Unfortunately, high blood pressure does not cause symptoms, so the condition may remain unrecognized for decades as it slowly raises the risk of stroke, kidney failure and heart attack. Lowering high blood pressure through lifestyle choices and drugs saves lives, yet only one in six people with hypertension has blood pressure under control. (Once you've been diagnosed with hypertension you are classified as "hypertensive" thereafter, even if your blood pressure is brought under control.)

Measuring Blood Pressure

The standard method of measuring BP involves inflating a blood-pressure cuff (a *sphygmomanometer*) around the upper arm while listening at the front of the elbow, over the brachial artery—a branch of a branch of a branch of the aorta. The air pressure inflating the cuff is higher than the pressure within the artery, and temporarily stops blood flow into the arm. As the cuff is slowly deflated, at some point the pressure in the brachial artery surpasses the pressure in the cuff, reestablishing blood flow. This point is heralded by a "whoosh" of blood that can be heard when a stethoscope is placed over the artery. The pressure at which this sound is heard indicates the *systolic* blood pressure—the pressure as the heart contracts. The *diastolic* pressure—the pressure as the heart relaxes—is the level at which the sound can no longer be heard. When blood pressure is reported as, for example, 120/80 (120 over 80), the top number is systolic and the bottom number is diastolic. (The numbers refer to mm Hg, or millimeters of mercury—a pressure measurement based on how high a certain pressure will raise the mercury column in a mercury barometer.)

Normal Numbers

Normal blood-pressure levels are based on the measurements of thousands of people. These levels allow doctors to predict complication rates based on different measurements. For example, the risk of stroke in a seventy-year-old man with a BP of 180/70 is much higher than that of his identical twin with a BP of 120/80. Although healthy BP is generally below

140/90, there is no particular number that defines normal blood pressure. Recently, an American blood-pressure working group called JNC-VII defined any number between 120/80 and 140/90 as indicating "pre-hypertension," meaning that even these lower values may raise the risk of cardiovascular disease. A BP of 90/60 may be perfectly normal for some people. Lower blood pressure readings are especially common in young women.

Blood pressure varies during the day. It is lowest at night, during sleep, and rises during the day, but it may vary from moment to moment. If you are resting, your BP may change from 120/80 to 125/75 in seconds. During periods of either emotional or physical stress, BP may vary more widely. For example, systolic blood pressure should always rise during exercise, while diastolic should either drop marginally or stay the same.

A marked rise in BP during exercise is associated with chronic (long-term) hypertension. Since a normal, healthy

Hot tubs

What could be more relaxing than immersing yourself in a vat of scalding water? For those undeterred by the risk of second-degree burns or bacterial super-infection, hot tubbing is an excellent pastime. Relaxing jets of bubbling water are soothing but have no other therapeutic value. Posted above most commercial hot tubs is a sign warning of the risks to people with hypertension. Is this fact or folly?

There is no clear evidence that a hot tub will raise your blood pressure. In one hot tub study (researchers were taking a break from trying to cure cancer), people with and without hypertension were cajoled into a hot tub for ten minutes. (Recruiting volunteers for this type of trial is not very challenging.) Blood pressure and heart rate were measured throughout the study. The results showed that systolic blood pressure dropped and heart rate rose during immersion, and returned to normal after ten minutes on dry land. Those signs above hot tubs may be to protect the hot-tub owners from liability suits—like those warning labels on coffee cups announcing that the contents are hot.

person's blood pressure should be below 140 systolic and 90 diastolic, hypertension exists if either of these numbers is higher. A newly recognized medical decree calls for even lower blood pressure in those with diabetes—less than 130 diastolic and less than 80 systolic.

Signs and Symptoms
Hypertension dramatically increases the risk of other diseases, such as strokes, heart attacks and congestive heart failure (see Chapter 7). It is also the most common cause of kidney failure requiring dialysis. Most hypertension is called *essential hypertension*, a cryptic medical phrase meaning "it exists because it exists, and we don't know why." Doctors do know that there is a marginal genetic component; having a hypertensive parent doubles your risk. However, it isn't well understood why some people develop hypertension while others remain free of it. A recent study of 2,600 people suggested that the greater a region's concentration of air pollutants (like sulfur dioxide), the higher people's blood pressure was likely to be. However, this represents a negligible contribution to the incidence of hypertension. It has also been shown that the highest incidence

Defining high blood pressure

Category	Systolic (mm Hg)	Diastolic	Risk of dying
Optimal	below 120	below 80	
Normal	below 130	below 85	
High-normal	130–139	85–89	
Hypertension			
Stage I	140–159	90–99	double
Stage II	160–179	100–109	triple
Stage III	over 180	over 110	very high

Based on information from the National High Blood Pressure Education Program

of hypertension in North America is found among those of African descent.

The most common form of hypertension is *isolated systolic hypertension*: the systolic number is above normal while the diastolic is fine. You should not take solace in having only systolic hypertension, as this too is associated with cardiovascular complications.

The dilemma of hypertension lies in its silence. Although many people are convinced they can feel when their blood pressure is high, there are no reliable symptoms. If hypertension is very severe, it can cause headaches and even strokes. However, headache is such a common and non-specific symptom that it is difficult to attribute it to elevated BP. The condition is most often discovered through a BP test during a physical with your family doctor.

Exposure to chronically elevated blood pressure gradually damages the walls of the arteries, the way a busy road becomes covered with potholes. A frayed artery is more likely to suddenly clog up and become blocked, creating a heart attack or stroke.

The good news about hypertension is the treatment available, through both medications and other means. Medical intervention can prevent many of the potential complications of high blood pressure.

Hypochondria and Munchausen syndrome

It is not unusual for people to avoid physicians. Those who enjoy visits are often called hypochondriacs. Hypochondriacs steadfastly believe they have serious medical problems despite assurances based on the absence of objective support. Feelings of fear and preoccupation must be present for at least six months before the label can be properly applied. Munchausen syndrome is a disorder named after Baron Karl H. Munchausen (1720–1797), an author of fabulous and exaggerated adventure stories about his travels. People with Munchausen syndrome deliberately harm themselves or others for attention.

Evidence of Damage from High Blood Pressure
A number of factors in your health or your medical history may also suggest to your doctor that you have a problem with chronic hypertension.

Heart
- left ventricular hypertrophy (a thickened heart)
- congestive heart failure (CHF)
- angina (pain related to arteriosclerosis)
- previous heart attack
- previous coronary angioplasty
- previous bypass surgery

Arterial
- aortic aneurysm (a ballooning of weak arterial wall)
- peripheral vascular disease (due to narrowings of the arteries to the legs)

Brain
- stroke
- transient ischemic attack (TIA), a quickly resolving stroke

Eyes
- retinal involvement causing blindness

Kidneys
- kidney dysfunction and/or kidney failure

White-Coat Hypertension
Emotional stress raises blood pressure, so when BP is measured by a physician it can be falsely elevated. This phenomenon is called white-coat hypertension—a reference to the stress some people experience when they visit the doctor. Accordingly, you

may be treated for a condition that only exists when you see your doctor.

White-coat hypertension should be suspected when you have normal blood pressure readings outside the doctor's office, no organ damage despite an apparent history of chronic mild hypertension and an apparent lack of response to blood-pressure medications. White-coat hypertension is more common in women. It is rarely the cause of severe hypertension (over 200/110).

The solution to white-coat hypertension is not to avoid doctors but, rather, to invest in a home blood-pressure machine, which can cost from $50 to $150 U.S. A home BP machine is also useful for ascertaining your response to BP therapy.

The BP cuff must fit around your upper arm, just as it does at the medical office. Digital, wrist and forearm cuffs are poor alternatives and may produce inaccurate readings. To avoid falsely elevated numbers due to the fear of discovering hypertension, readings should be documented over months.

Blood pressure machines come in three types: mercury, aneroid and automatic. The standard, mercury, is used in most doctors' offices. The aneroid is lighter and more portable but is also delicate and prone to damage, and fixing it requires precise factory work. The automatic units are ideal for home use. They are easy to operate and the digital display is easy to read. However, they too can be fragile, and they must be periodically checked for accuracy.

It is important not to be obsessive about documenting your blood pressure at home. Some people take five to ten measurements per day, when one is sufficient. Before taking your BP, ensure that the cuff fits properly around your upper arm. If the cuff is too small, the blood pressure will be falsely elevated; if the cuff is too large, the blood pressure will appear falsely low. Also, relax and be quiet; when you talk while your

Ambulatory BP monitoring

Ambulatory blood pressure monitoring is another way to document BP in a normal environment. This test involves wearing a computerized blood pressure cuff that inflates and measures your blood pressure up to seventy-five times in twenty-four hours. The test costs less than buying a home blood-pressure machine.

blood pressure is being measured, there is a slight but potentially important rise in systolic BP, an average of 7 mm Hg.

Your blood pressure readings should be taken, faxed or e-mailed to your doctor's office for review at each appointment. As well, bring your home monitor along to the doctor's office to verify its accuracy.

Causes of Hypertension

Approximately 3 percent of the time, there is a clear cause for hypertension. The causes include excessive alcohol consumption, valvular problems such as a leaky mitral or aortic valve, steroid use, kidney disorders and numerous other conditions. Although, for most people, a cause cannot be identified, screening tests are necessary to examine urine, kidney function, red blood cell count, blood electrolytes (including potassium, chloride and sodium) and heart function (*electrocardiogram*).

There are other, more expensive tests, but they diagnose rare conditions and are not part of routine screening. These tests, which include special imaging investigations like CAT scans and ultrasounds, are reserved for certain conditions in which a specific cause is suspected. For example, a hypertensive person with a *bruit* (audible blood flow when a stethoscope is placed over a blood vessel) in the abdomen may be referred for a more specific test that diagnoses renal artery stenosis—narrowing of the kidney (renal) arteries. Because this condition is rare, not everyone is routinely tested for it.

Some secondary causes of hypertension
• kidney disease
• renal (kidney) artery stenosis (narrowing)
• coarctation (congenital narrowing) of the aorta
• Cushing's syndrome (excess production of steroid)
• primary hyperaldosteronism (excess production of the hormone aldosterone)
• pheochromocytoma (an adrenaline-producing tumor)
• hyperthyroidism (overactive thyroid gland)
• certain drugs

As well, certain people require more extensive investigations. These include those with hypertension at a young age (younger than thirty-five) and those with uncontrolled BP despite taking numerous anti-hypertensive drugs.

An often unrecognized contributor to hypertension is medication and other drugs. Anti-inflammatory drugs (NSAIDs), steroids (drugs such as prednisone, used for numerous diseases, and anabolic steroids, taken by athletes and others) and cocaine are a few examples.

Treatment of Hypertension

Too often, physicians don't have time to counsel their patients adequately about the benefits of lifestyle modification. Studies have demonstrated that people are interested in, and are capable of, changing unhealthy pursuits, although it may take them numerous attempts before they succeed. There are a number of non-drug treatments for lowering blood pressure, summarized by the acronym SWEAR:

- Salt restriction
- Weight reduction and nutrition
- Exercise
- Alcohol restriction
- Relaxation

Salt Restriction

S is for salt restriction. Sodium is an element (its symbol is Na, from the Latin *natrium*). Sodium combines with chloride to form sodium chloride, or common salt (NaCl). The terms "sodium" and "salt" are often used interchangeably in references to dietary intake, but it's worth remembering that they are not really the same thing.

Salt restriction works for some people but not all. This is a controversial recommendation, since empirical evidence of its effectiveness is sparse. A recent study showed that older people who reduced their salt intake were more likely to normalize high blood pressure without medications. The strategy was less successful for younger people. A North American diet often includes five to ten times the amount of sodium required by our bodies. Efforts to lower dietary salt are complicated by the fact that most of it is ingested in processed

Sodium content of some popular foods (in milligrams)

canned tuna (3 oz/90 g)	300
lean ham (3 oz/90 g)	1,000
one egg	65
Swiss cheese (1 oz/30 g)	75
Cheddar cheese (1 oz/30 g)	175
cottage cheese ($\frac{1}{2}$ cup/125 mL)	450
canned vegetables ($\frac{1}{2}$ cup/125 mL)	50–500
bread (one slice)	150
bagel ($\frac{1}{2}$)	200
shredded wheat cereal (3/4 cup/175 mL)	less than 5
cooked rice ($\frac{1}{2}$ cup/125 mL)	less than 10
cooked pasta ($\frac{1}{2}$ cup/125 mL)	less than 10
fruit (any form)	less than 10
salad dressing (2 tablespoons/25 mL)	200–400
salted peanuts ($\frac{1}{4}$ cup/50 mL)	200
potato chips (1 cup/250 mL)	250
soya sauce (1 tablespoon/15 mL)	1,000
canned soup (1 cup/250 mL)	1,000

Decoding salt labeling

- *No Salt Added:* no salt is added during food processing
- *Reduced Sodium:* 25 percent less sodium than the regular type of the food
- *Light in Sodium:* at least 50 percent less sodium than the regular type of food
- *Low Sodium:* less than 140 mg of sodium/serving
- *Very Low Sodium:* less than 35 mg of sodium/serving
- *Sodium Free:* less than 5 mg of sodium/serving

---

foods. Only 25 percent of the salt in an average diet is added at the table.

A problem with studying salt restriction is the difficulty in gauging compliance. Unless people are videotaped twenty-four hours a day, how can a researcher be sure they are not secretly stuffing themselves with salted bagels, pretzels and cans of soup? A low-sodium diet is about 2,400 mg (2.4 grams) of sodium per day (contained in 6 grams of salt). Because salt is composed of sodium and chloride, 2.4 grams of sodium is not the same as 2.4 grams of salt. Talking about salt as a weight is meaningless for most people.

Sodium content is listed on the packaging of most foods, but it can be deceiving unless you check the serving size. For example, a 50-gram bag of potato chips (a poor source of nutrition) may claim a sodium count of only 300 mg, but the fine print may show that this applies to a 10-gram serving— only a few chips. If you multiply this by five, you'll find that the sodium content of the whole bag is 1,500 mg—most of a day's worth of a low-sodium diet.

Weight Reduction and Nutrition
W is for weight reduction. Obesity increases the risk of many diseases, including hypertension, diabetes, certain forms of cancer, gallstones, respiratory disorders and overall mortality.

The conclusion that obesity is associated with an increased likelihood of illness should be published in the *Journal of the Obvious*, alongside the story that using a cellphone while driving or driving immediately after the Super Bowl increases the chances of a car accident. Every 10 pounds (4.5 kg) of added weight results in an average 4 mm Hg increase in systolic blood pressure. Lose that excess weight, and your blood pressure will drop along with those unwanted pounds. However, your body must be overweight for weight loss to reduce your BP; if a thin person loses weight, the BP stays the same. For those with an obesity problem, a 10-pound weight loss has a similar effect to taking anti-hypertensive medication on lowering BP.

On paper, weight loss is easy. Reduce the calories you take in by eating less, and increase the calories you expend with a regular exercise program. However, the multibillion-dollar weight loss industry is an indication that the perfect body weight is harder to achieve than it seems.

For resistant cases of obesity, prescription drugs are available, including orlistat (Xenical) and sibutramine (Meridia). Orlistat interferes with the action of a stomach enzyme (lipase) that breaks down dietary fat; instead of losing weight by eating less, people on orlistat shed pounds because fat digestion and absorption are inhibited. Orlistat can reduce weight within two weeks. The mean weight loss after six months of treatment is just over 12 pounds (5.4 kg).

The side effects of this drug can be annoying. When dietary fat remains undigested in the gastrointestinal tract, it comes out the other end. Depending on how much there is, this undigested fat may cause abdominal bloating, excessive flatulence (is there another kind?), diarrhea and oily stools. About 9 percent of patients who try orlistat need to stop the drug due to the side effects. Patients on orlistat are prescribed supplements of the fat-soluble vitamins (A, D, E, K and beta-carotene), since the body's absorption of these vitamins is reduced by the drug.

Sibutramine was approved for use in the United States in 1997 and in Canada in 2000. It prolongs the effects of natural chemicals in the brain that regulate appetite, resulting in appetite suppression. This drug has been shown to reduce weight by 5 to 10 percent after six months of use. Uncommon but serious side effects include high blood pressure and rapid heart rates. In March 2002, the sale of sibutramine was halted in Italy after fifty reports of side effects.

Nutrition can also have a strong impact upon blood pressure. For example, you can lower your blood pressure by eating foods high in potassium. Moderation is important, though, because high levels of potassium in the blood can be very dangerous, especially to those with kidney disease. Foods rich in potassium include bananas, peaches, apricots, prunes, fruit juices, milk, spinach, fish, pumpkins, potatoes, beans (such as green and lima) and squash.

A low intake of calcium may be associated with higher blood pressure, although this connection has not been proven. The same may be true of magnesium. Sources of magnesium include leafy green vegetables, beans and nuts.

In the recent DASH study (Dietary Approaches to Stop Hypertension), three diets were studied. The first was the typical North American diet, high in animal fats and fast food. The second was the same diet with fruits and vegetables added. The third was the DASH diet, which is low in bad fats (saturated fats, cholesterol) and high in fruits, vegetables, grains, fiber and low-fat dairy products. The amount of sodium in each diet was the same (about 3 grams per day). This study showed that the second diet was more effective than the first, and the third diet was most effective in lowering blood pressure.

The higher the individual's BP, the greater the anti-hypertensive effect of the DASH diet. These results prove that adhering to simple, healthy nutritional choices will help maintain normal blood pressure and reduce unnecessary drug dependency. Unfortunately, many doctors do not take the time or have the knowledge to dispense proper nutritional advice.

Exercise

E is for exercise. Working up a sweat for a minimum of thirty minutes a day five days a week will lower blood pressure, independent of weight loss. Exercise is good for cardiovascular health; people who exercise regularly are 70 percent less likely to develop hypertension than their sedentary neighbors. Unfortunately, only a small percentage of the North American population regularly gets off the couch and into the gym.

Sweating for thirty minutes a day isn't very complicated; you don't need someone with a kinesiology or physical education background guiding you around the gym. However, tai chi, yoga and stretching are not exercise. They may be beneficial in their own way, but they do not even approach the benefit of running, swimming, aerobics classes, exercise bikes and other continuous workouts.

Exercise means spending at least thirty minutes working until you are increasingly short of breath and sweaty from moving large muscle groups repetitively. Run, swim or hike, play squash or basketball or ride a bike. Unless you are too infirm to partake, it is useful to get your heart racing. Studies have clearly demonstrated the benefits of regular exercise in reducing blood pressure and lowering the risk of cardiovascular disease. However, if you are not accustomed to working out, begin gradually— and if you have doubts about your health, consult your physician first. (See also "Stress Testing" in Chapter 3.)

The precise benefit in reducing blood pressure is difficult to gauge in an individual, but studies show an average of approximately 10 to 14 mm Hg systolic reduction and 7 to 8 mm Hg diastolic reduction with regular exercise. Reductions in BP are observed after about three months of exercise, and you will experience the full benefit after about six months. After that, it is important to keep moving. When laziness takes over, your blood pressure will gradually drift higher again. Loss of interest results in loss of benefit.

Alcohol Restriction

A is for alcohol restriction. Alcohol overuse may account for 10 percent of cases of hypertension. Intake beyond one standard drink a day (equivalent to 12 grams of alcohol) is associated with higher BP levels and stroke risk. To put this in a weekly perspective, recommendations call for no more than fourteen drinks per week for men and nine for women. These drinks should not all be consumed in the same sitting. (Because they have smaller livers and the liver breaks down the alcohol, as a general rule women should drink less than men. As well, more frequent alcohol use in women has been linked to a higher risk of breast cancer.)

Just over 5 percent of North Americans indulge in more than two drinks of alcohol per day. This creates more than a hang-

---

What's a drink?

All of the following are considered "one drink" and have approximately the same alcohol content:

- a 5-oz (142 mL) glass of wine (12 percent alcohol)
- a 12-oz (341 mL) bottle of beer (5 percent alcohol)
- a 1.5-oz (45 mL) shot of liquor (40 percent alcohol)
- a 3-oz (90 mL) glass of sherry or port (18 percent alcohol)

over risk; alcohol is filled with non-nutritional calories, hence the term "beer belly"—although, in fact, all forms of alcohol are associated with excess calories and weight gain. And weight gain will further contribute to hypertension and heart disease.

Several studies have indicated that a modest alcohol intake could actually keep the heart healthier. This effect is not fully understood, but it has something to do with alcohol's ability to raise HDL, the good cholesterol. However, these positive effects do not keep increasing with the number of drinks consumed. While intoxication increases with the amount used, health benefits plateau at two drinks. There may be beneficial "anti-oxidant" properties in alcohol, but this suggestion is speculative.

Alcohol abuse is a cause of congestive heart failure, although only 10 to 15 percent of alcoholics develop severe heart failure. There is thought to be a genetic susceptibility that singles people out for this unfortunate but self-directed fate.

Relaxation
R is for relaxation. Relaxation techniques, including yoga and transcendental meditation, are associated with lower blood pressure numbers. Bookstores have sections devoted to relaxation techniques. Unfortunately, acupuncture, herbs and spices do not promote blood pressure reduction.

Drugs
Years ago, it was discovered that lowering blood pressure pharmacologically (with medication) dramatically reduces the incidence of strokes and heart attacks. Anti-hypertensive medication, available since 1958, saves lives. These drugs are discussed in Chapter 10. As with all pills, there may be side effects; however, the benefits far outweigh the risks. Unfortunately, many people are "non-compliant" about taking pills: they take them erratically, remembering one day and forgetting the next.

This is a particular problem with hypertension, since the condition does not often produce symptoms. In order to avoid complications, it is important to take anti-hypertensive medication regularly. Most are prescribed to be taken once per day, to improve compliance.

It is rare to achieve blood pressure control with one drug (monotherapy), especially for elderly people. More than 60 percent of those with hypertension need more than one drug to reach their target blood-pressure levels, and in many cases the blood pressure is poorly controlled despite two or three medications. Causes for this may include poor compliance and poor lifestyle choices.

Cholesterol

The word cholesterol strikes fear in few. There is a tacit acknowledgment of its association with heart disease, but people are often too complacent to learn about cholesterol and the heart.

Cholesterol is a fat (*lipid*) found in the membranes that surround our cells. It is integral to normal body structure and function. However, high levels of cholesterol in the blood are associated with narrowed arteries. The higher the blood cholesterol, the greater the risk of narrowing.

To ensure a steady supply, the liver makes cholesterol even if we don't consume any. This internal production explains why some people can't budge their blood cholesterol levels despite obsessive attention to diet. They may be consumed by their desire to avoid "second-hand" cholesterol, but their bodies go on manufacturing it unless the liver is surgically removed. Many people are genetically programmed to maintain high cholesterol values, and require medication to reduce them.

There is a reported case of a man possessed by a psychiatric disturbance. Believing his liver to be the source of his discontent, he studied surgical textbooks and skillfully operated on himself. He was sidelined by the unexpected pain caused by knifing his way into his own abdomen and lifting up the liver (he used a clever array of mirrors to guide him). The surgeons on call at the hospital marvelled at the skill he displayed in his misguided attempt at a hepatectomy. Liver removal should only be undertaken in the hands of skilled professionals, and is not recommended to lower cholesterol.

Cholesterol can't move through the body on its own. It doesn't dissolve in blood, but it's carted about in cholesterol "dumptrucks" (*lipoproteins*) along the blood superhighway. The evil dumptruck, LDL (low-density lipoprotein), picks up cholesterol from the liver and unceremoniously dumps its load into arteries, including the coronary arteries. Arteries that are impregnated with cholesterol become narrow, and it is this narrowing that can lead to angina and heart attacks. The good dumptruck, HDL (high-density lipoprotein), also motors along, but it carries cholesterol from the arteries back to the liver, where it is chewed up and transformed into bile acids, which aid digestion. People with high levels of the good cholesterol (HDL) and low levels of the bad cholesterol (LDL) have the lowest incidence of coronary artery disease.

Measuring cholesterol

In the United States, cholesterol is measured in milligrams per deciliter (mg/dL). Under the global system of SI (système internationale) units, however, it's measured in mmol/L, or moles per liter. (In this context a mole is not a small, fuzzy rodent, but convenient shorthand for an extremely large number of molecules—6.23×10^{23}.)

To convert mmol/L of HDL or LDL to mg/dL, multiply by 39—or divide mg/dL by 39 to get mmol/L. To convert triglycerides, use a factor of 89.

Normal Cholesterol Values

The level of cholesterol considered acceptable depends on the presence or absence of other cardiac risk factors. An acceptable LDL level for a seventy-year-old woman after bypass surgery is different from the level considered acceptable for a twenty-five-year-old with no history of cardiovascular problems. If you are concerned about coronary artery disease, you should know your cholesterol profile and your optimum targets. To obtain your cholesterol profile, you must have a blood test to measure your total cholesterol, LDL, HDL and *triglycerides*, another type of fat. The next step is to tally your cardiac risks. If you have already had heart disease (heart attack, angioplasty or bypass surgery), the number of cardiac risks becomes irrelevant. The risks are:

- hypertension
- diabetes
- tobacco use
- family history
- HDL below 0.9 mmol/L
- age over forty-five for men
- age over fifty-five (under fifty-five if post-menopausal) for women

The more risk factors you have, the lower your LDL should be. If you have a history of angina, heart attack, angioplasty, bypass surgery or coronary artery disease, your LDL should be under 2.5 mmol/L and your HDL should be higher than 0.9 mmol/L, regardless of how many other risks are present.

The most important recent study was the five-year Heart Protection Study (HPS), published in 2002. Involving more than twenty thousand British patients, the HPS included a number of sections, one of which randomly assigned patients to take either simvastatin or a placebo. (Simvastatin is one of the statin drugs, which lower the lipid levels in the blood; a placebo is an inert "sugar pill" used for comparison.) Unlike most other large drug trials, the HPS was conducted independently, without financial support from a pharmaceutical company. Previous studies of cholesterol treatment had included narrow groups of patients; HPS studied a wider population.

The patients in the study had an average total cholesterol level of 5.9 mmol/L, and an average LDL of 3.4. Those who received simvastatin had significantly fewer heart attacks and strokes over the course of the study, and required heart surgery and coronary angioplasty less often. HPS is the first trial to show that lowering cholesterol can reduce stroke risk. Although the patients had various levels of LDL cholesterol, the risk reduction was very similar. Even those with LDL levels below 2.6 benefited from taking simvastatin. Moreover, during the five years of the trial, the placebo group and treatment group continued to separate, meaning that the longer the drug was used, the greater the benefit became.

HPS showed that anyone with diabetes, prior coronary disease (a heart attack, bypass surgery, coronary angioplasty or angina), a stroke, carotid artery narrowing, leg artery narrowing or untreated hypertension (in men over sixty-five) benefits from cholesterol-lowering with statin treatment, regardless of his or her original LDL cholesterol level. This is truly a landmark trial.

Assessing Your Risk

Most people want a fairly clear estimation of their heart-attack risk. To calculate this risk, physicians may use a combination of history, physical exam and specific investigations such as stress testing. They may also use a point system to calculate the ten-year likelihood of coronary artery disease in people not known to have diabetes or heart disease. The questionnaire below is based on the Framingham Table, developed in Massachusetts. Points are based on risk factors, and the tally at the end indicates your risk of suffering a heart attack.

How Old Are You?

Pick the one correct answer here, and add the corresponding points to your risk factor.

	Men	Women	
• 30–34	–1	–9	
• 35–39	0	–4	
• 40–44	1	0	
• 45–49	2	3	
• 50–54	3	6	
• 55–59	4	7	
• 60–64	5	8	
• 65–69	6	8	
• 70–74	7	8	Score _____

What Is Your Overall Cholesterol Level (in mmol/L)?

	Men	Women	
• Below 4.14	–3	–2	
• 4.15–5.17	0	0	
• 5.18–6.21	1	1	
• 6.22–7.24	2	2	
• Over 7.25	3	3	Score _____

What Is Your HDL Cholesterol Level (in mmol/L)?

	Men	Women
• Below 0.9	2	5
• 0.91–1.16	1	2

	Men	Women	
• 1.17–1.29	0	1	
• 1.30–1.55	0	0	
• Over 1.56	–2	–3	Score _____

What Is Your Systolic Blood Pressure (in mm/Hg)?

	Men	Women	
• Over 160	3	3	
• 140–159	2	2	
• 130–139	1	1	
• 120–129	0	0	
• Under 120	0	–3	Score _____

Do You Smoke?

If you are a smoker, add 2 points.   Score _____

You should now have five separate scores. Add them up to get your total risk factor. To determine your percentage risk of having coronary artery disease in the next ten years, look up your risk factor in the appropriate table.

Men

Points	Risk	Points	Risk
1	3%	8	16%
2	4%	9	20%
3	5%	10	25%
4	7%	11	31%
5	8%	12	37%
6	10%	13	45%
7	13%	14	Over 53%

Women

Points	Risk	Points	Risk
1	2%	10	10%
2	3%	11	11%
3	3%	12	13%
4	4%	13	15%
5	4%	14	18%
6	5%	15	20%
7	6%	16	24%
8	7%	17	Over 28%
9	8%		

Diabetes Mellitus

Diabetes mellitus is a complex disorder of insulin character-ized by elevated blood sugar levels. Insulin is a hormone secreted by the pancreas, an organ that resides at the back of the upper abdomen. Insulin fits into the membranes of the body's cells like a key into a lock, causing an influx of glucose— the sugar carried through the blood—into each cell.

Someone with diabetes mellitus has either a deficiency in insulin production, or a resistance to the action of insulin. In type I diabetes (formerly called insulin-dependent diabetes), the body has an insulin deficiency because cells of the pancreas have been destroyed. This may be an autoimmune disorder in which the body attacks and destroys its own cells—in this case, cells in the pancreas, called the islets of Langerhans. The destruction may also result from an abnormal response to an otherwise benign viral infection. Type I diabetes is usually diagnosed in children, and accounts for 10 percent of all cases.

In type II diabetes (formerly called non-insulin-dependent diabetes), insulin levels may be elevated, as the cells resist insulin's action. Type II diabetes usually develops after age forty, and is responsible for the remaining 90 percent of diabetics. About 80 percent of type II diabetics are overweight, and there is a genetic predisposition to its development.

When insulin is either lacking or ineffective, the level of sugar in the blood rises. Called *hyperglycemia,* this condition damages the lining of blood vessels, and increases the chance of developing atherosclerosis of major arteries, including the coronary arteries. Sugar is excreted in the urine, as the body tries to flush out the excess. *Polyuria* (excessive urination) occurs with high blood sugar, and leads to excessive thirst (*polydipsia*), a common symptom of diabetes.

Historical references to diabetes have been identified in writings thousands of years old. Diabetes was named by a physician in ancient Greece and means "siphon." The disease is called "mellitus," Greek for "honey," because of the sweet taste of the sugar-laden urine. Descriptions of urine, including color, taste and turbidity (cloudiness), were considered an important diagnostic tool by physicians for centuries. Fortunately, the folly of these claims has led to their demise as a pseudo-diagnostic tool. Unfortunately, other alternative practices have not accompanied urine tasting into the medical dustbin.

Diabetes increases the risk of cardiovascular disease, including heart attacks and strokes, by up to fivefold. It is the most common cause of heart attacks in people under age thirty, and someone with diabetes is significantly less likely to survive a heart attack. Unfortunately, diabetes is likely to be associated with other major cardiac risk factors, which dramatically raises the likelihood of a heart attack. People with diabetes are much more likely to have high blood pressure and high cholesterol levels than their non-diabetic neighbors. Therefore your target levels of blood pressure and cholesterol must be much lower if you have diabetes.

Obviously, diabetes is not a good thing. But diabetes can be controlled through a combination of diet, exercise and medications. Medications may take the form of pills or daily insulin injections. Keeping blood sugar levels as normal as possible, reduces the chance of coronary artery disease.

There are many excellent books on diabetes written by endocrinologists (diabetes experts). Cardiologists do not treat diabetes, but they adjust the risk profile of a diabetic cardiac patient to reflect the implications of the disease.

Obesity

Obesity—defined as weight more than 30 percent above "ideal body weight"—increases the chance of other risk factors, including diabetes, high cholesterol and high blood pressure. In addition, obesity is in itself a risk factor for cardiovascular disease, because excess weight puts a strain on the heart.

Body weight can be measured in a number of ways. It is sometimes discussed in terms of body mass index (BMI), which relates height to weight. A man who is five feet tall (1.5 m) and weighs 200 pounds (90 kg) has a BMI of nearly 40; a man of the same weight who is six foot three (1.9 m) has a BMI of 25. A BMI between 25 and 30 indicates overweight; a BMI over 30 indicates obesity.

Hormone Replacement Therapy

It is rare for a widely used and trusted therapy to take a 180-degree turn after more careful study, and be banished to pharmaceutical hell. But it happened to hormone replacement therapy (HRT), in the form of combination estrogen and progesterone pills. HRT has been used by blissfully unaware women (and the occasional man trapped in the wrong body) to combat the symptoms of menopause for decades.

Menopause occurs at an average age of fifty-one. It's a body-altering event that causes women to lose their natural childbearing potential as their ovaries stop pumping out eggs. This loss of reproductive ability is noted in very few mammalian species; most continue to bear young into old age. As levels of the hormones estrogen and progesterone drop, various physical and emotional symptoms may result.

The symptoms of menopause are myriad, but are significant in only one-quarter of women. Hot flashes and night sweats are the most common symptoms, and almost invariably respond to hormone supplements. Without HRT, hot flashes and night sweats may take one to two years to resolve, and may persist much longer.

Other symptoms of menopause include vaginal dryness and painful intercourse, both of which benefit from topical estrogen cream. (*Topical* treatments, such as creams, are applied directly to the area affected.) Some women suffer from urinary incontinence, which does not tend to improve with topical therapy. After menopause, osteoporosis accelerates and bone loss increases the risk of fractures.

As well, women's previously low risk of heart disease rises after menopause. After a few more decades, their risk of coronary artery disease approximates that of men. One explanation for this phenomenon is that there are nearly twice as many women aged seventy-five and older, as by that time many men have died from heart attacks. It had been observed, however, that women taking hormone replacement therapy were less likely to have coronary artery disease than those not taking it. With so many purported benefits, it is no wonder HRT was the most commonly prescribed medication in North America.

Could the observed reduction in heart-disease risk be explained by other factors? Did women on HRT simply live healthier lifestyles than their hormone-less sisters? Were women on HRT in a higher income bracket, which is associated with a longer life-span? What theories could account for the apparent benefit of HRT?

We know that HRT has a beneficial effect on cholesterol levels. After natural menopause, LDL rises and HDL drops. HRT reverses this trend, offering a ready explanation for the lower risk of CAD. But while HRT was all the rage, it had never been tested in an organized, prospective randomized way. When such studies were finally undertaken, the results shocked doctors, women and drug companies everywhere.

The first whiff of doom was aired by HERS (Hormone Estrogen Replacement Study), a study conducted in the United States. HERS was a "secondary prevention" trial, since the women enrolled had evidence of coronary artery disease. Nearly three thousand women were randomly assigned to receive either estrogen and progesterone or a placebo. Because so many patients were involved, the two groups were nearly identical in all other respects; any difference in results could not be attributed to one group having a greater number of smokers, more people with large feet or big-footed smokers. The women were monitored for an average of four years.

The study showed that within the first year, the women on estrogen and progesterone were more likely to die of heart disease (with smoother, younger-looking skin, however), although this trend disappeared after four years. This shocking result suggested that these supplemental hormones should not be used in women with a previous heart attack or other evidence of coronary artery disease. Further, women taking estrogen and progesterone had a higher incidence of leg blood clots (*deep venous thrombosis*, or *DVT*), blood clots in the lungs (*pulmonary emboli*, or *PE*) and gallstones. The study found no significant difference in breast cancer rates, a dreaded fear of many women.

The next nail in the HRT coffin was the Women's Health Initiative, a trial designed in 1992. Part of this study was terminated earlier than planned due to the important interim results.

This complex trial involves 160,000 post-menopausal women between fifty and seventy-nine years of age, and encompasses various areas of study. One arm of the study randomly assigned women who had had a hysterectomy to take either estrogen alone (progesterone is not needed after a hysterectomy) or a placebo. Another arm of the study, including nearly 30,000 women, assigned them to take either estrogen plus progesterone or a placebo. The estrogen used was called premarin, because it derived from pregnant mares' urine. The study was "double-blind"—neither the women nor the researchers knew whether any specific woman was on supplemental hormones or the placebo, so their expectations could not affect the results. In 2002, the estrogen and progesterone arm of the trial was terminated after five years of follow-up, because there was an excessive number of breast cancer cases and cardiovascular events (including heart attacks, strokes and pulmonary emboli) in the group receiving the combined hormones.

Whereas the risk of death from heart disease began returning to normal after the first year, and the risk of blood clots rose quickly after the women began the hormones, the excess number of breast cancer cases developed after three to four years of hormone replacement therapy. Accordingly, it was

---

The Women's Health Initiative

For one section of this study, 8,500 women were treated with HRT (estrogen and progesterone) and 8,100 were given a placebo. The women on HRT suffered a higher rate of numerous problems. It was calculated that among 10,000 women treated with these hormones per year, there would be:

- seven more heart attacks
- seven more strokes
- eight more blood clots in the lungs
- eighteen more blood clots in the legs
- eight more cases of breast cancer

judged that prolonged exposure to estrogen and progesterone is necessary to increase the risk of breast cancer.

The HRT group did have fewer cases of colon cancer and hip fractures, but this benefit was outweighed by the increased risk to the women's hearts and breasts.

With the announcement of the termination of this arm of the Women's Health Initiative, jaws dropped throughout the medical and pharmaceutical world. Whereas small retrospective studies had once suggested cardiovascular benefits with HRT, a large, well-done and definitive trial has proven the opposite, at least for women using combination estrogen and progesterone. It appears that HRT with estrogen and progesterone should be avoided in post-menopausal women, as it does much more harm than good. Women with bothersome symptoms of menopause should be dissuaded from pursuing this treatment due to the greater likelihood of dying as a result. Women already taking these drugs should not have their prescriptions renewed.

It took a large, well-conducted trial to provide a definitive answer to the HRT question. The results are a testament to the necessity of investigating drugs thoroughly before espousing their use. If the alternative medicine industry had the same concern about health as those that designed this study, society would be spending far less money on unproven remedies, including dubious herbal menopause remedies. People who rely on advice from untrained or suspect sources expose themselves to serious risks.

Novel Risk Factors

In addition to the risk factors for coronary artery disease already discussed—smoking, hypertension, high cholesterol, diabetes, family history, male gender and increasing age—there are also risk factors that are less dangerous on their own but increase the effects of the more established risks. Examples are obesity, a sedentary lifestyle and, perhaps, personality type.

In addition, there are less familiar risk factors that have only recently been identified and studied. These risks include high levels of homocysteine, Lp(a), C-reactive protein and other factors. Treatment options have yet to be evaluated; trials may involve tens of thousands of patients and take many years. But since 30 percent of heart attack patients have no traditional significant risk factors (aside from age and sex), we may find that these newly identified risks have a strong influence on coronary artery disease development.

Homocysteine

Homocysteine is one of twenty different amino acids, which are the building blocks of all proteins. We all have homocysteine coursing through our veins and arteries, but high levels may predispose us to atherosclerosis. The issue is a complex one, and the contribution of high homocysteine levels to coronary artery disease remains to be clarified. It is possible that only those with very high levels are truly at increased risk.

High levels of homocysteine are most often found in men and are more common in:

- people with kidney disease
- those with high-protein diets
- those who use caffeine excessively
- those who smoke
- people with certain rare diseases.

Thus, carnivorous male smokers who drink a lot of coffee and have weak kidneys are at the greatest risk.

B vitamins and folic acid (folate) lower homocysteine levels in the blood, but they do not necessarily lower the cardiovascular risk. In 1998, the United States began to add folic acid to wheat flour. This move increased the population's daily intake, which in turn lowered homocysteine levels. The vitamin industry has capitalized handsomely on the association between folate B vitamins and homocysteine. However, there has yet to be a controlled study of the benefits of folic acid and/or vitamin B_{12} and/or vitamin B_6 in reducing cardiovascular risk by lowering homocysteine levels in the blood. Natural sources of folic acid include vegetables, tomatoes, citrus fruits and grain. A balanced diet rich in fruits and vegetables is (as we have all heard countless times) superior to and cheaper than well-marketed pills.

Screening everyone for elevated homocysteine levels would be expensive and unnecessary, especially since studies of the connection are inconclusive. Younger people (perhaps fifty or forty years old) who have coronary artery disease but do not have traditional risk factors, or those with a family history of premature heart disease, should have a homocysteine test. If the levels are found to be elevated, they may try the unproven strategy of using vitamin B_6, vitamin B_{12} and folic acid. For the time being, the balance of people with heart disease should simply pay attention to their overall diet.

Lp(a)

Lp(a) is a lipoprotein, a cholesterol-containing molecule that is very similar to LDL, only smaller. It carries a substance that may promote blood clotting, thus increasing the chance of a heart attack. As with homocysteine, high levels of Lp(a) have been associated with a higher risk of heart attack. However, other studies have failed to confirm this conclusion.

There is no indication that testing people for Lp(a) is useful. Laboratories don't even perform the test the same way. Further, there has never been a study involving treatment of high levels of Lp(a). Because Lp(a) levels are so tightly linked to LDL levels, it is questionable whether Lp(a) is truly a separate risk.

C-Reactive Protein (CRP)

CRP was first discovered in 1931 by Oswald Theodore Avery (1877–1955), a Canadian physician and immunochemist famous for his work with DNA. (He proved that it was not a protein that was responsible for transferring genetic information, as had been believed, but rather DNA.) CRP levels rise acutely in response to infections and illnesses, but their relation to heart disease would not be studied for another fifty years.

These days, CRP is an up-and-coming marker of heart-attack risk. When an artery becomes inflamed, as a result of cigarette smoke, high blood pressure, diabetes or high cholesterol, atherosclerosis results and plaques develop. CRP levels then rise as an indicator of the inflammation.

There is very good evidence that as the CRP level becomes higher, the risk of a heart attack increases. A recent study concluded that CRP is better at predicting cardiovascular risk than LDL. But because there is no accepted treatment for elevated CRP, it is difficult to justify routine screening. The American Heart Association does not recommend widespread screening for CRP. (CRP levels are measured in milligrams per liter, or mg/L. A level of less than 1.0 mg/L is considered low, 1.0 to 3.0 mg/L is average and anything above 3.0 mg/L is elevated.)

Our knowledge about traditional risk factors has advanced our understanding and treatment of heart disease. Unfortunately, we continue to look at the problem with blurred vision. Novel risk factors such as homocysteine, CRP and Lp(a) may sharpen our visual acuity in the future, further expanding our ability to predict and treat cardiovascular disease.

3. Cardiac Testing

Imagine that you live in an apartment building, on the thirtieth floor. You love to watch the sun rise as you eat breakfast, with an unimpeded view of the horizon. (Hopefully, that breakfast is a bowl of granola with skim milk and a piece of fruit, and not an egg McMuffin and hashbrowns.) With the first thrust of winter you retreat to the warm Florida sun for the rest of the season. Tanned and slightly heavier, you return to your apartment. In the morning you open the blinds to find that your panoramic vista of the city has been usurped by a condo directly across the street. You start to feel a pressure in the center of your chest that you have never experienced before. It's mild but you also have numbness in your left arm and fingers.

After ten anxiety-filled minutes, the pressure in your chest begins to ebb. You sit on your favorite chair and stare at the concrete, pondering whether to call your building superintendent, your doctor or your spouse. You quickly decide not to worry your spouse (a common mistake) and that the superintendent is unlikely to tear down the condo. Worried you will be found dead in your favorite chair overlooking the condo, you focus on this unusual pressure. As you try to convince yourself that you have strained a muscle golfing or carrying luggage, an inner voice tells you that there is another explanation. You concentrate on your chest and realize, with relief, that the pressure has completely gone. You are frightened but back to normal.

A few weeks later, seeing your doctor about another matter, you decide to mention this brief scare. Your doctor suggests that you may have had an episode of *angina*—not an actual heart attack, but a warning that you are at serious risk of a heart attack. You protest that you feel fine now, but your doctor warns you that you can't ignore angina. You must get a definite diagnosis, and probably treatment. You are referred to a cardiologist. After taking your history and giving you a physical examination, the cardiologist will perform an electrocardiogram in the office and consider further investigations.

The Electrocardiogram (ECG)

ECGs have been around since the late 1890s and were invented by a Dutchman named Willem Einthoven. In 1924, three years before his death, he was awarded a Nobel Prize in physiology and medicine for his discovery. (ECGs are sometimes called EKGs, from the German *Elektrokardiogramm*.) He was not in very good company during that decade, as other Nobel prizes were awarded for suspect work. For example, two years after Einthoven, in 1926, Dr. Johannes Fibiger was recognized for the discovery of a parasite called spiroptera carcinoma, which he claimed was the cause of all cancers. In 1927, Dr. Julius Wagner von Jauregg was given the Nobel Prize when he claimed he could cure dementia by inoculating patients with malaria. In 1949, Egas Moniz was honored for his "discovery" that lobotomies cured some psychoses. It has taken the Nobel Committee some time to ensure the prize is awarded for truly brilliant work.

As with most seminal discoveries, Einthoven's work would have been impossible without a multitude of discoveries in numerous other fields. Science is like a pyramid. Advancement doesn't occur in a vacuum, but is built upon the investigations of others. The peak is never reached, as more and more is discovered.

An ECG is a simple and cheap method of evaluating many aspects of heart function. Electrical impulses originate in a special portion of the heart, the sino-atrial node, and course through the muscle in a wave of electricity. This electrical energy triggers the heartbeat, or muscle contraction, that propels the blood. The electricity can be detected and measured by electrodes attached to the arms, legs and chest, and translated into a tracing called an electrocardiogram.

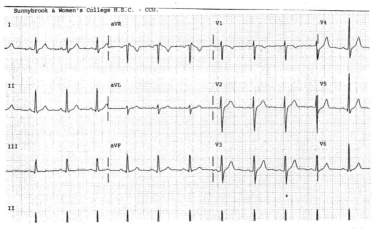

An ECG records the electrical activity of the heart on a scroll of paper. Each of the ECG's twelve leads (I, aVR, V1, etc.) traces activity from a different vantage point, so the spikes and bumps differ from one tracing to another.

An ECG is a rapid and non-invasive test that provides accurate diagnostic and life-saving information for a long list of important cardiac problems. For example, the most serious types of heart attacks are diagnosed primarily by particular abnormalities on the ECG. All disturbances of heart rhythm are diagnosed by ECG, including those that are dangerously fast and those that are dangerously slow.

The electrocardiogram is essentially a screening test. It gives us a piece of the whole cardiac picture, but only occasionally—as in an acute heart attack or rhythm disturbance—the definitive piece. Like all tests, it has limitations and pitfalls. It must be interpreted within the context of these, which requires expertise and experience.

Some heart problems may go undetected by the ECG. Someone who has had a prior heart attack may develop a normal electrocardiogram over time. Some parts of the heart may not be electrically visible on the ECG; even during an acute heart attack, an ECG may appear normal. Many people ask about their ECG, perhaps under the impression that a normal ECG means a healthy heart, but a normal ECG can hide a heart problem, just as apparent abnormalities may simply indicate variations of normal. With an ECG, shades of gray are common; it is like viewing scenery without your eyeglasses. Other, more detailed, expensive and time-consuming tests evaluate heart function more completely. However, the information gleaned from an ECG in proper hands is always useful.

Stress Testing

More than seventy years ago, it was discovered that monitoring an ECG during exercise provides useful diagnostic and prognostic information about coronary artery disease. Thus was born the field of exercise stress tests. The person being tested exercises on a treadmill, while hooked up to a computer, and the computer provides an ongoing ECG.

The treadmill was invented in the early nineteenth century by Anthony Cubitt, a British civil engineer. Its initial application was in the British penal system, as a form of punishment, before it was outlawed as inhumane. This fact may not be surprising to those who perform on modern versions. Treadmill testing was first used to evaluate coronary artery disease in 1928. A stress test is performed under the supervision of a technician and a physician. Treadmills are a desirable mode of exercise, but some laboratories insist that tests be done on exercise bikes instead. Stress machines—like cars, microwaves and most consumer items—come in a variety of shapes and sizes, from low-end models to fancy systems costing upwards of $40,000 U.S.

A stress test is simple, non-invasive (no needles or probes) and inexpensive, with very low risk for the patient.

Indications for Stress Testing

Stress tests are ordered for a variety of symptoms. Any patient with chest pain or shortness of breath (*dyspnea*) out of proportion to the degree of exercise needs a stress test. These symptoms may indicate angina; however, symptoms alone are rarely diagnostic of coronary artery disease and supporting evidence is required. Because heart disease can be fatal, early diagnosis is important. Indeed, anyone with a tiny nibble of chest pain, shortness of breath, palpitations, lightheadedness or even diarrhea may be referred for a stress test. But you should not assume you have heart disease just because you are having this test. Most people who undergo stress testing have a normal result.

Some people who complain of exertional shortness of breath perform so well on the test that the likelihood of heart or lung disease causing their symptoms is remote. Casting such a wide net into the stress testing sea creates potential problems related to the stress tests's reliability. Like an electrocardiogram, stress testing may indicate a problem where none exists. It can also miss serious coronary disease. Therefore, the interpretation of a stress test is both a science and an art, requiring careful evaluation of many pieces of information.

Exercise stress tests are also used to screen people at high risk for heart disease, even if they have no symptoms. This high-risk group includes those with a worrisome risk factor such as smoking, high cholesterol, diabetes and high blood pressure. Even without symptoms, people at high risk should have a screening exercise test prior to embarking on an exercise program. Treadmill testing is a good reflection of exercise capacity; if your test results are normal, it's probably safe for you to undertake the exercise program.

The Test
Your stress test requisition will advise you to wear comfortable clothing, which should be self-evident. Arriving in a cocktail dress and high heels, especially if you are male, will make the test more difficult. Most people get quite warm during exercise, so light summer clothing and a good pair of walking shoes or sneakers are a good idea. The technician will connect you to an ECG that is monitored on a computer screen during the test. An ECG tracing can be generated on paper as needed, with the push of a button. Your blood pressure and heart rate will be measured frequently. It is common for the starting blood pressure to be mildly elevated, possibly because of anxiety about the test. Anxiety may also explain an elevated heart rate at the beginning of the test; nobody likes to see doctors and nobody likes tests. However, high readings at the start of the test may also point to a cardiovascular problem. The correct explanation is not always clear.

During the test, the treadmill elevates and the speed is simultaneously increased, in stages three minutes apart. This means that you will be walking up a steeper and steeper incline, faster and faster. This increase follows a standardized computer protocol—commonly the Bruce protocol, first reported by Dr. Robert A. Bruce in 1956—which allows the doctor to compare exercise times among large groups, and helps in interpreting the results.

The test is called a stress test, not a relaxation test, because it is designed to stress you to the point of reproducing your symptoms. You should only stop running when you feel you cannot continue, or when the physician stops the test.

Results of the Test

Many factors are used to interpret a stress test. Although some results are very abnormal (a positive test) or entirely normal (a negative test), interpretation by a specialist is required. It may be difficult to exclude coronary artery disease with 100 percent certainty based on an exercise stress test alone, but the test can still be extremely useful. It's cheap and quick, with instantaneous results, and it's an excellent screening tool for determining whether more aggressive testing is warranted.

The amount of time spent on the stress test is important, as there is a direct relationship between exercise time and cardiac prognosis. An inability to complete stage I (less than three minutes) is a bad prognostic sign. The ability to exercise beyond stage IV (more than twelve minutes) is a good prognostic sign; even people with coronary disease who exercise beyond twelve minutes on a Bruce protocol have less than one chance in a hundred of dying from cardiac disease in the ensuing year. The longer you can exercise, the firmer the doctor's conclusions are likely to be.

Cathy grimaced as another sharp pain bit into her left shoulder and chest. Like every other episode of the past month, it stopped within seconds. She arose from her chair, put down her book and paced around her bedroom.

A forty-eight-year-old account executive, Cathy was active and healthy. When she had begun experiencing these unusual chest pains, about a month ago, her doctor had attributed them to menopause. The pains came both when she was at rest and during her treadmill routine.

Only five years ago, at age sixty-four, her father had suffered a heart attack. He had survived but had been left with chronic shortness of breath and occasional bouts of angina. So Cathy often worried about her heart.

Cathy had never smoked. Her blood pressure, blood sugar and cholesterol were all perfect. She couldn't understand why this pain had entered her life. The following day she contacted her family doctor, who arranged for a stress test.

On the day of the stress test, Cathy climbed the two flights of stairs to the lab. Dressed in her tracksuit, she stepped onto the treadmill, where the technician connected her to the ECG. At first Cathy trotted with little effort, staring at the blank white wall in front of her. After three minutes the speed and height of the treadmill increased, but her breathing remained easy and controlled as the test continued. At six minutes, when the settings increased further, her breathing became more labored and she started to sweat.

"Doing all right?" the doctor asked as she checked Cathy's blood pressure. "Any pain or difficulties?"

"No problem," replied Cathy, by now running.

The technician was monitoring the ECG on the computer screen. Every three minutes, the machine spat out a hard copy of the ECG tracing. "Everything looks fine so far," the technician reassured Cathy.

The treadmill continued, increasing its pace every three minutes. After twelve minutes Cathy was having trouble keeping up. After twelve minutes and forty-seven seconds, she asked the technician to stop. The machine slowed to a halt and Cathy was led to a gurney and asked to sit. Her vital signs (pulse, blood pressure, breathing) were monitored. The doctor scanned the ECG tracings, and reviewed the blood pressure and heart rate recordings generated during the test.

From the cardiologist's point of view, the results were definitive. "It looks perfectly normal," she told Cathy. "I'll send a full report to your doctor, but based on these results, with this degree of exercise, your pain is not from your heart."

"Then what is it from?" Cathy asked.

"Well, I'm not sure. I can tell you what it isn't, but I can't be sure what it is. You'll have to go back to your GP and sort it out with him."

Cathy continued to complain of intermittent chest pain for years, and she underwent more tests, but no cause was ever identified. She worried less each time a cause was ruled out.

Only a small percentage of people complaining of chest pain have coronary artery disease. Women with chest pain are much less likely to have heart disease than men. In many cases, no cause of chest pain is ever identified. As a general rule, the longer a person experiences symptoms such as chest pain without a diagnosis being established, the less likely it is that a serious medical problem exists. Significant illness, including heart disease, is typically progressive; it cannot be ignored for long.

Heart Rate and Blood Pressure

The way your blood pressure and heart rate respond to the exercise of a stress test is called the *hemodynamic component* of the test. Heart rate should always increase during stress testing. Your target heart rate is the minimum acceptable rate to confirm that your test result is negative. If you stop exercising after reaching a heart rate of only 100, even without symptoms or changes on the ECG, the test is likely inconclusive and the doctor cannot be sure this is a normal result; there is no way of knowing whether an abnormality would have surfaced at a heart rate of 110 or 120.

Your target heart rate during exercise represents 85 percent of the maximum heart rate predicted for your age group. This can be calculated by subtracting your age from 220. For example, a sixty-year-old has an age-predicted *maximum* heart rate with exercise of 160 (220 – 60). The *target* heart rate during stress testing, 85 percent of 160, is 136 beats per minute. Once this heart rate is reached, the treadmill result is more valid. Recently, modifications of this age-dependent formula have been proposed, as research suggests that it underestimates maximum heart rate in older people and overestimates it in younger ones. A more accurate equation for age-predicted peak heart rate is 208 – (0.7 × age), which is a bit harder to calculate in your head. However, regardless of which peak is used, if you quit the test while your heart is well below it, the test is inconclusive.

Sometimes people are unable to reach their target heart rate because of drugs they are taking. Commonly used cardiac medications may lower the resting heart rate and slow its rise with exercise, which limits the amount of work the heart performs, and thus reduces the frequency of angina. Anti-angina pills, including beta-blockers and some calcium channel blockers, work both ends of the "supply-demand" equation: they increase blood flow through the coronary arteries, and decrease demand by "restraining" the heart. These drugs may be safely withheld for forty-eight hours prior to the test, to improve the accuracy of the results. But don't stop taking your medication without checking with your doctor.

Systolic blood pressure (the top number) normally rises with exertion while diastolic blood pressure (the lower number) decreases. If the systolic blood pressure fails to rise during exercise, this may indicate serious heart disease, because it suggests that the heart is not receiving enough blood through the coronary arteries to generate a higher blood pressure. One caveat is the anxiety factor. A person may be so nervous prior

What's your target heart rate for a stress test?

| | Old system | | New system | |
Age	Maximum	Target	Maximum	Target
20	200	170	194	165
25	195	166	191	162
30	190	161	187	159
35	185	157	184	156
40	180	153	180	153
45	175	149	177	150
50	170	144	173	147
55	165	140	170	144
60	160	136	166	141
65	155	132	163	139
70	150	127	159	135
75	145	123	156	133
80	140	119	152	129

to the test that blood pressure rises before the treadmill is even switched on. As the test begins and anxiety fades, the exercise-induced rise in blood pressure may be the same as the anxiety-related increase, resulting in an apparently flat blood pressure response with little change from beginning to end.

Symptoms during the Test

You may experience chest pain while performing an exercise stress test. However, such pain is only one piece of the puzzle, and may be the least significant; symptoms are less important than other indicators measured on the test, such as exercise time, blood pressure, heart rate and ECG tracings. If these other indicators are normal, symptoms are of little value in analyzing the results.

The physician's goal is to tire you out during the exercise test. You *should* develop shortness of breath and fatigue; if you don't, the exercise was inadequate. A common error is to stop the test abruptly when the target heart rate is reached, but the target heart rate may vary by 15 percent, so achieving this rate is not a reason to terminate the test. If there are no changes on the ECG, and no blood pressure or heart-rate concerns, treadmill testing should be symptom-limited. In other words, the test should be stopped when fatigue and shortness of breath or some other symptom make it too difficult to continue.

The Electrocardiogram in Stress Testing

The most important part of a stress test is the electrocardiogram. Changes on the ECG, known as ST segment depression, are a clue to the presence of coronary artery narrowing. The type and amount of ST segment depression are very important. Changes in the heart rhythm may also occur, but are less frequent.

A fundamental problem with treadmill testing is the "gray zone." It has been known for decades that stress testing can give false positive and false negative results. Some people with completely normal coronary arteries develop ST segment depression on the ECG during exercise. Only more advanced testing proves that the stress test was misleading. Equally

---

About your stress test

The goal of a stress test can be thought of as climbing a hundred steps to reach a mountain peak, with the risk of tumbling at each step. How far you climb determines how the test is reported. If you fall off—that is, the ECG shows significant changes—the test is positive. Where you fall off determines how strongly positive it is. If it happens within the first twenty steps, severe heart disease is present. If it happens after the eightieth step, the disease is likely minor. If you stop early, without plummeting (without ECG changes), interpreting the stress test can be difficult; perhaps abnormalities would have developed if the ascent had continued. If you stop on the ninety-fifth step, however, chances are very good that you do not have coronary disease—or, if you do, that it is very minor.

Risks of stress testing

As with every medical procedure—every action in life, for that matter—the risk is not zero. Whether you are having an appendectomy, taking penicillin, driving a car or brushing your teeth (especially while driving), you are taking a risk. In stress testing, your risk of complications depends on your age, the presence of serious heart disease and the presence of other diseases. Clearly, a twenty-five-year-old marathon runner has a lower chance of suffering a heart attack on the treadmill than an eighty-five-year-old diabetic with kidney failure, lung cancer and one leg. On average, there is one chance in ten thousand of a serious complication during a stress test of someone with heart disease, and much less risk for someone with a healthy heart. That's why stress tests are generally performed under the supervision of a physician as well as a technician. However, the greatest risk occurs when a person with suspected heart disease fails to undergo the test.

common, and potentially more serious, some people with coronary artery disease have an apparently normal stress test. Because of the gray zone, it is vital that all the different aspects of the stress test, including exercise time, blood pressure, heart rate, symptoms and changes on the ECG, be evaluated together, for the most accurate interpretation possible.

In properly selected individuals, stress testing is a very useful screening tool. People with a very low likelihood of disease are commonly referred for a stress test. In these cases, a "positive" result may be ignored as incorrect. Alternatively, if the likelihood of coronary artery disease is very high, then it would take a perfect result, normal in all respects, to obviate the need for further testing. The test is most appropriately done on people with an intermediate likelihood of coronary artery disease, since they will benefit most from the screening.

Perfusion Imaging

You may also have treadmill testing in conjunction with *perfusion imaging*, a combination that significantly improves the test's accuracy in diagnosing heart disease. Prior to treadmill testing, your doctor inserts an intravenous (IV) line through which a drug can be injected. The drug (thallium or hexamibi) is selectively absorbed into the heart muscle, and it is "tagged" with a very small amount of radiation—less than that present in a chest X-ray. A special machine takes pictures of the heart and measures the amount of radiation it emits. The pictures indicate in what part of the heart muscle the drug has settled.

Perfusion imaging offers an added layer of information to regular treadmill testing and can diagnose a previous heart attack. If you have suffered a heart attack, part of your heart muscle is dead. Because that part is no longer receiving blood, it cannot absorb the radioactive drug, so there will be no radioactivity in the dead part of the heart. Imagine the heart as a river with five streams branching off, each emptying into a separate lake. If neon orange dye is dumped into the source of the river, the lakes will all turn orange. If one of the streams is blocked, however, the lake at its end will not change color.

Perfusion stress tests can do more than diagnose a past heart attack. They can also show areas of the heart at risk of a future heart attack. This goal is accomplished by injecting the drug and taking pictures before exercise, when normal heart muscle is literally bathing in blood. These resting pictures are compared to pictures taken after the drug is injected during peak exercise. With exertion, parts of the heart supplied by narrowed arteries don't receive enough blood. Therefore, only a small amount of the drug gets through. Compared to the pre-exercise (rest) images, the exercise picture looks like a doughnut with a bite taken out of it. Since this indicates a narrowed artery and a risk of heart attack, the cardiologist may order an *angiogram* to examine the blood vessels directly.

Some people are unable to do a treadmill test—perhaps because of orthopedic problems like hip and knee trouble, or because they are too ill. In these cases, a drug called dipyridamole (Persantine) is injected for a Persantine stress test. This drug replaces the exercise portion of the test, but stresses the heart in a similar way. Side effects include nausea, lightheadedness, headache, chest pain and, rarely, heart rhythm disturbances, but all these are usually brief and self-limiting. If they are more serious, an antidote to dipyramidole called aminophylline is available in the stress lab.

Stress testing, in its many forms, is a valuable and easily accessible investigative technique. Stress tests are excellent screening tools to assist in diagnosing coronary artery disease, and they will likely remain an important part of our diagnostic toolkit in the future.

Echocardiography

Echocardiograms, also known as cardiac ultrasound or echo, have dramatically revolutionized the diagnosis of heart disease in the past few decades. Prior to the advent of echo, cardiac ailments were diagnosed mainly through physical examination skills by doctors. The ability of clinicians to recognize subtle findings of heart disease, though often impressive, remains limited. Because abnormalities are often absent in the early stages of severe heart disease, many conditions were not diagnosed until they were advanced. Late diagnosis results in late treatment, which often leads to a late patient.

Echocardiography leapt into clinical practice in the 1970s. Modern machines provide wondrously detailed information about cardiac anatomy and function; they can show weakness of the heart muscle, heart-valve abnormalities and anything else that is structurally wrong. (At a cost of $250,000 to $300,000 per machine, the pictures had better be good!) Every cardiac patient should undergo this procedure.

Echocardiograms are painless, safe and non-invasive. A technologist slides a hand-held probe (transducer) lubricated with gel over the patient's chest wall. The transducer emits high-frequency (ultrasound) sound waves that safely penetrate the chest wall and heart. The sound waves reflect back to a receiver in the transducer, which translates them into a two-dimensional image of the heart, which is recorded as a digital image or onto a VCR tape.

Electron Beam Computed Tomography (EBCT) Scan

German engineer Wilhelm Roentgen discovered X-rays in 1895. The first published X-ray image was of his wife's left hand. Roentgen elected not to seek proprietary or patent rights for his discovery. In 1901, he won the first Nobel Prize awarded in physics.

A conventional medical X-ray is a beam of energy directed at the body. In computed tomography (a CT scan), the X-ray moves around the body in a circle, allowing multiple views of the same anatomy. With this advanced technology, there is less radiation exposure than from a single conventional X-ray image.

Ultrafast CT scanning is faster than a regular CT scan and therefore results in very detailed images of the heart. These scans can detect calcium deposits in the coronary arteries that may indicate atherosclerosis. Unfortunately, ultrafast CT offers no functional information about the heart. It does not eliminate the need for a conventional stress test or perfusion scan, and it offers less vital information than these non-invasive techniques. These quick scans are important diagnostic tools for many diseases, but coronary artery disease is not one of them.

Ultrafast CT scans for the heart have cropped up in clinics across the United States, and many people have been sucked into the machine, literally and figuratively. But claims that ultrafast CT scans add to your doctor's understanding of your cardiac risk should be met with skepticism. If you are a candidate for an ultrafast CT, you are also a candidate for an inexpensive stress test, which will offer much more useful information. And if you do choose the quick scan, an abnormal result will mean that you need a stress test anyway.

Magnetic Resonance Imaging (MRI)

The first MRI on a human was done in 1977, in a machine nicknamed Indomitable. Since that time, this complicated technology has progressed rapidly. An MRI machine is a giant magnet that, in combination with radio waves, rearranges our water molecules and records the energy released as they return to normal. This released energy is translated into breathtaking, detailed images of the human body.

The magnetic pull of an MRI machine is so powerful that it can suck your watch right off your wrist. All metal must be kept out of the MRI room, including dental implants and pacemakers. Surgical clips (unless they are in the brain) and orthopedic hardware are fine, because they are firmly embedded in the body.

Cardiac MRI provides much more detailed images than echocardiography. Because echocardiography is cheaper and more widely available, cardiac MRI is used to complement the information from echocardiography, rather than replace it. In the ensuing decades, as cheaper, faster and more portable MRI systems become available, MRI will replace our present imaging technology.

4. Coronary Artery Disease and Heart Attacks

The most common form of heart disease involves the coronary arteries. As mentioned in Chapter 1, arteries are thick-walled blood vessels that transport oxygen-laden blood to the head and body. Veins are thin-walled blood vessels that return blood to the heart before it is pumped to the lungs for oxygen replenishment. The heart muscle depends on blood flow through the coronary arteries, and any interruption, however brief, can carry dire consequences.

Atherosclerosis

Arteries can become narrowed by a disease process called atherosclerosis. Like a five-lane highway reduced to one lane, a narrowed coronary artery will not allow enough blood through, which will restrict the oxygen supplied to the heart muscle.

Atherosclerosis is not a modern problem; it has been identified in Egyptian mummies (and daddies). The disease begins

Arteries and atherosclerosis

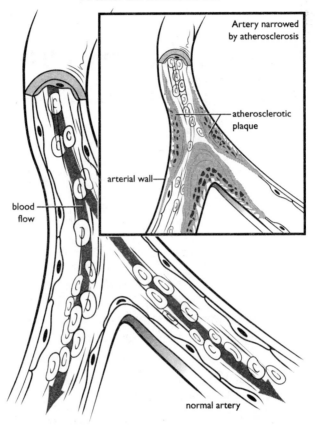

early, but manifests later in life. When the insides of the arterial walls are injured in some way, there is an inflammatory response; inflammation is the body's reaction to nearly all injuries. The inflammatory process is complex; different kinds of blood cells rush to the scene of the "accident" to repair the injured blood vessel. During the repair, some cells remain and are integrated into the repair job. This process attracts fat, which migrates into the walls of the arteries. The injury typically recurs, just as car accidents tend to recur at an intersection without a stop sign. Although the body is doing its best to repair the damage, repeated episodes of inflammation cause the blood vessel to narrow. Atherosclerosis involving the coronary, cerebral (brain) or renal (kidney) arteries is responsible for nearly half of all deaths in North America. The other top causes of death include cancer, accidents and homicide.

What causes these injuries to the blood vessels? The answer to this question is not completely known. Injury is a common occurrence in people with high cholesterol, high blood pressure and diabetes, and in people who smoke. Controlling these risk factors will reduce inflammation and prevent atherosclerosis from developing or progressing. There are probably other factors involved as well.

Angina

Angina is both a symptom and a diagnosis. It occurs when two conditions are met: one or more of the arteries is narrowed by atherosclerosis, and the body's demand for blood is higher than normal—perhaps when you're walking up a hill, or screaming at the kids at the top of your lungs, or walking with your kids up a hill and screaming at them. In these situations, the body needs more blood to function, and demands more from the heart. The heart itself also needs more blood, so that it can pump faster and harder. If atherosclerosis has narrowed the heart's supply lines (the coronary arteries), the needs of the heart and body cannot be met, and angina occurs as a warning symptom.

Angina versus heart attack

A heart attack—and the symptoms it produces—results from complete blockage of blood flow through a coronary artery, while angina results from insufficient blood flow through the artery. Patients who suffer from angina may have enough blood squeezing through the narrowing when the body is at rest, but the demands of physical exertion can rarely be met. The symptoms of angina are often a warning to slow down.

The history

When you tell your physician about a medical problem, his or her first task is taking a history. This provides an opportunity to listen to your complaints in your own words, and to establish understanding and trust, even though you may be nervous and intimidated. Some histories take a few minutes, others an hour, depending on the condition. Someone complaining of chest pain may need a lengthy history to sort out the problem. Someone with a sore throat may not require as long an interview (unless the throat is so sore that speech is impossible). Some doctors are skilled at establishing trust, while others may unknowingly alienate the patient, resulting in mistrust. Some people provide good histories, while others are unable to verbalize their problem clearly. Language or cultural barriers often complicate the process. Since an unclear history can make diagnosis and treatment tricky, people unable to communicate with the physician due to a language barrier are at a significant disadvantage, even when an interpreter is available. A person with chest pain from simple acid indigestion may be led down the path of cardiac investigations and even treatment for angina, because the history is unclear.

Angina does not necessarily feel like the classic chest pressure people associate with heart attacks. Although often described as central and left-sided chest pressure, akin to a weight on the chest, angina may be sharp or dull, burning or squeezing, pushing or pulling. It may be felt in the middle of the chest, on the left side or right side, in the shoulder, arm, fingertips or elsewhere. Some people feel their angina as shortness of breath, and have no chest discomfort at all. One patient complained of left earlobe pain whenever he walked quickly, which resolved with rest; upon investigation, he was found to have severe coronary artery disease. So it's important not to disregard symptoms and attribute them to indigestion or a strained muscle. All concerns should be discussed with your physician. Self-diagnosis can be dangerous.

Many people deny their symptoms out of fear of what they may represent. It is not uncommon to hear "It's just a pulled muscle" or "It's only very mild pain." These shouldn't be your last words. Doctors (and spouses) are on the lookout for the heart attack itself, but it's common for people to have a few days of warning symptoms prior to a serious or fatal heart attack. This is why it's so important to have symptoms checked early.

In most cases, angina first appears during exertion. In a person accustomed to regular exercise, the angina may begin twenty minutes into a thirty-minute treadmill routine. In a more sedentary individual, angina may be precipitated by taking out the garbage, walking up stairs or shovelling snow.

In everyone, angina begins suddenly. One day you have no symptoms and the next day chest pressure starts. This is deceptive, leading many people to believe that their heart condition has just begun. In fact, the opposite is true. Although the manifestations of atherosclerosis come on suddenly, the narrowing of the arteries develops over decades. Early atherosclerotic disease is present in children and progresses gradually, hastened by genetics, smoking, high cholesterol, smoking, high blood pressure, smoking and, of course, smoking. Autopsy studies of young soldiers killed in Korea and Vietnam showed early stages of coronary artery disease.

A narrowing of a coronary artery may not cause angina, even in a person accustomed to regular exercise, until it blocks about 70 percent of the artery's channel. This is because coronary arteries have a property known as *coronary flow reserve*. During normal resting conditions, a clean, open artery has five times more blood flowing through it than the heart requires. Thus a significant degree of narrowing can develop before there is less blood flow than the heart needs. As the fat-filled area continues to encroach on blood flow, however, angina eventually develops.

Steve, a sixty-two-year-old lawyer, was awakened at two in the morning by a dull ache in the center of his chest. Assuming he had indigestion, he sat at the side of the bed and tried to belch, but the pain persisted. He made his way to the kitchen slowly and quietly, so as not to awaken his wife, and poured himself a glass of milk, but the feeling only intensified. He was certain he had heartburn from last night's lasagna; he thought he could taste the tomato sauce repeating on him. He had had a similar feeling two weeks earlier, starting in the middle of a squash game at the club. Sweaty and spent, he had experienced an ache in the center of his chest after an unsuccessful lunge at the ball. That time, he'd shrugged off the pain and it had gradually ebbed. Since then he had experienced daily episodes of chest heaviness whenever he exerted himself.

Steve made his way to the study and sat in his favorite chair, wondering what he should do. He looked nervously at the telephone, but he was paralyzed by indecision. Then, just ten minutes after awakening him, the ache began to subside. He touched his chest. The sensation was gone.

For hours after he returned to bed, Steve tossed, obsessing about his wife and his three young kids, about his business and his frantic life. He slept briefly, anticipating pain that never came. Deep down, he knew it wasn't indigestion.

At seven a.m., Steve called his secretary and asked her to cancel his morning appointments. He kissed his wife goodbye, and appeared unannounced at his family doctor's office. He'd gotten lost trying to find his way there; it had been that long since his last visit. Had it been two years or three? For two hours he thumbed through magazines, waiting to hear his name, while the patients around him were called one at a time. Finally, it was his turn. After a brief history and physical examination, the harried physician pronounced his verdict.

"I think you're suffering from angina," he explained. "Here's what we'll do. I'll give you a prescription for nitroglycerin spray. The drug can cause a headache, but it will help the angina. If the symptoms recur, spray it under your tongue. If the pain is severe, or doesn't resolve after three sprays, get yourself to hospital, okay?" Steve nodded. He was numb, but ready to get dressed and go to work.

"One more thing," said the doctor. "You need a stress test. I would prefer to do it sooner rather than later. Make an appointment with my secretary on the way out, and I'll see you in follow-up after the stress test to review the results. Lay off the squash games until we sort this out. I don't want you having a heart attack on the court."

Steve did poorly on the stress test, and was sent for an angiogram. It indicated that he had significant coronary disease. He underwent a successful angioplasty to reopen two narrowed blood vessels. Then he tackled his lifestyle; he cut back on his cigars, reduced his workload and began to follow a strict diet recommended by his dietitian.

Steve's choices may have saved his life. Despite the temptation to convince himself that his symptoms were nothing, he faced up to the possibility that there was a serious problem with his heart. After a few weeks of denial that could have cost him his life, he dealt with the problem sensibly and realistically.

Heart Attack

Angina occurs when blood flow through a coronary artery is significantly reduced, with some blood still squeaking by. A heart attack (*myocardial infarction*, or *MI*) occurs when blood flow through a coronary artery abruptly ceases. It's the difference between squeezing through a partially shut door and being locked out. When part of the heart muscle is deprived of blood and oxygen, it stops functioning. The longer it takes to reestablish the blood flow, the more heart muscle dies. The more heart muscle is dead, the more likely the patient will develop severe heart failure or die. Reopening the artery is the ideal treatment for a heart attack.

Heart attacks are sudden. They may occur during stressful periods, such as after an emotional outburst or the death of a loved one. But they also commonly happen in the early morning hours when the person is under no strain at all. Although they occur suddenly, it takes decades and decades of artery abuse to create the milieu for a heart attack. Coronary atherosclerosis develops slowly, during youth, into adulthood, middle age and onwards, so while it may appear that a heart attack was caused by a particular event, this perception is false. People who have angina or who have had a heart attack were, in effect, walking slowly toward the edge of a cliff. Although a stressful event may speed up their pace, without medical intervention their fall is inevitable.

Although a heart attack is preceded by progressive restriction of blood flow, due to narrowing of the coronary artery, it is caused by a blood clot that actually blocks the artery. First the narrowing creates an unstable environment inside the artery, like a gasoline spill waiting for a spark. When that spark arrives, a blood clot forms and obstructs what little blood flow is left. Even relatively minor arterial narrowing—of 40 to 50 percent—can abruptly close off, causing a heart attack.

Recognizing a Heart Attack

Symptoms of a heart attack are typically more severe than those of simple angina. People usually, although not always, know that something is amiss. They may feel pressure, stabbing, constriction or pain. Like angina, not all heart attacks produce pain on the left side of the chest and down the arm;

Possible signs and symptoms of a heart attack

Symptoms are what you feel yourself (such as pain); signs are what others see (such as paleness).

- pain, pressure or discomfort somewhere in the central body area (possibly in the arm and/or jaw)
- shortness of breath
- sweating
- nausea and/or vomiting
- anxiety

pain may be felt in the neck, arm, back, jaw or elsewhere. A heart attack may be accompanied by sweatiness, nausea or anxiety. Some people develop sudden shortness of breath, yet may have no chest pain or pressure. Ten percent of heart attack victims suffer a silent event, in which there are no symptoms at all—most often older people with diabetes. A previously unrecognized silent heart attack may become apparent during a routine examination, or when an electrocardiogram or cardiac ultrasound shows evidence of heart damage.

The period of greatest risk is during the first few hours after a heart attack; most deaths occur during this time. People who delay going to the emergency department, hoping their symptoms will disappear, are the most likely to die. If you think you are having a heart attack, chew an ASA tablet; the blood-thinning properties of the ASA may open up the blocked artery, and chewing the pill gets the drug into the bloodstream faster. Then call an ambulance. The psychology of delay is complex, but the risk of delay is great.

Diagnosing a Heart Attack

Heart attacks can be minor or major, depending on the area of artery that is blocked. In some heart attacks, the areas of damage are like niblets falling off an ear of corn; without

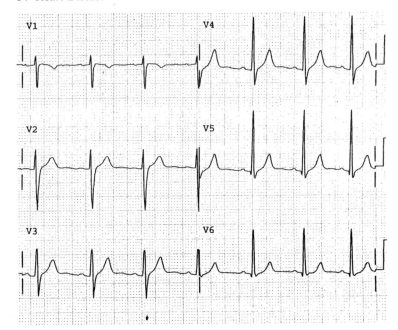

Compare the section of normal ECG, above, to the section below, which shows
an extensive heart attack. The diagnosis of heart attack is indicated by the broad,
rounded spikes, known as ST segment elevation.

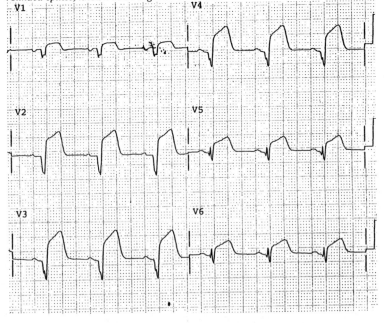

advanced diagnostic blood tests, these heart attacks may go unrecognized. When the heart cells die, they explode, and particles of the cells' contents are absorbed into the bloodstream. Blood tests can detect these particles and help diagnose the heart attack. It is like a million balloons filled with confetti; the more balloons burst, the more confetti there is to measure. The traditional measure of heart attack damage is a blood test for *creatine kinase* (CK), but sometimes the creatine kinase level is elevated when there is no heart damage, and sometimes it is normal when there is heart damage. A newer test that measures a substance called *troponin* is more reliable, being more sensitive and more specific for heart damage. The troponin test is more expensive, but it will soon render CK measurements obsolete. In either case, the higher the level—of troponin or of CK—the bigger the heart attack.

When someone comes to hospital with a suspected heart attack, one of the most important tests is an electrocardiogram (ECG). If the ECG shows ST segment elevation, then the treatment approach becomes more aggressive. If the ECG shows less specific changes, the amount of muscle damage is usually less and the treatment differs. If your doctor diagnoses a heart attack, one of the initial questions should be "Is there ST elevation on the ECG?"

When ST segment elevation is noted on the ECG, there are two treatment alternatives. There is increasing evidence that a primary angioplasty (see Chapter 5) is the quickest, most effective and best means of treating a heart attack patient who shows ST segment elevation. Unfortunately, most hospitals in Canada cannot offer this treatment, due to a lack of government funding and highly trained cardiologists. From a citizen's perspective, it seems reasonable for all of us to have access to this life-saving treatment at our local hospital. However, the

Canadian government ultimately decides how to ration health care. In the profit-driven U.S. health care system, on the other hand, cardiac services such as angioplasty are widely available at medical centers. While this may seem like a good thing, it means that expertise in cardiac care is diffused among many doctors. It is always advisable to seek out a doctor with vast experience in the procedure to be performed.

If angioplasty is unavailable, the next best option is thrombolysis. Special intravenous medications called thrombolytics are available at all hospitals, and represent the standard of care; they have been used to treat ST segment elevation heart attacks since 1985. A "thrombus" is a blood clot, and "lysis" means to destroy; a thrombolytic is a very powerful blood-thinner that destroys the blood clot.

Destroying the clot, either by squishing it out of the way through angioplasty or by dissolving it with a powerful clot buster, is the goal. Thrombolytics are either cheap (streptokinase costs a few hundred dollars) or expensive (TNK-tPA costs a few thousand). There are also new genetically modified products that are extremely expensive.

Thrombolytic therapy is mildly successful at opening a blocked artery. The earlier it is administered, the greater chance there is that it will work. Statistically, for every 1,000 heart attacks properly treated with a thrombolytic, thirty lives are saved. However, because they thin the blood, thrombolytics can cause a hemorrhagic stroke—serious bleeding inside the brain that is almost always fatal. For every thirty people saved from heart attack, there is one serious stroke. The survival benefit—thirty out of 1,000—may seem small, but with millions of heart attacks a year the survivors add up. Additionally, one might expect that patients would be spared serious heart damage when the artery is reopened, which may mean the difference between living with heart failure and living with a minimally damaged heart, although this has yet to be proven. An ASA tablet taken at the time of a heart attack, at a cost of pennies, saves an additional twenty lives per 1,000 patients treated.

After treatment is initiated, the duration of hospitalization depends on the severity of the heart attack. Every person requires *risk stratification*; that is, the patient cannot be discharged from hospital until the doctor has a sense of the risk of another heart attack. This assessment may involve exercise testing on a treadmill. Looking at the coronary arteries by injecting dye (an *angiogram*) has become a routine means of assessing future heart attack risk. The coronary angiogram determines whether further treatment with angioplasty, bypass surgery or medication is required. The jury remains out whether an angiogram should be customary for everyone who has had a heart attack, or whether only patients with high risk of heart attacks or positive stress tests, should undergo angiography. The decision to have an angiogram may depend as much on the hospital you are admitted to (does it have angiogram facilities?) as on the necessity for this invasive investigation. These factors can work against you either way: at a hospital that is not equipped to perform angiography, you may be less likely to have one if you need it; if the hospital does perform the procedure, you may be more likely to undergo one unnecessarily.

Angiogenesis

Angiogenesis is the development of small new blood vessels (capillaries) from pre-existing blood vessels; the word was first coined in 1935, in reference to the placenta. The process may be pathogenic (disease-causing), facilitating unimpeded growth of malignant tumors. It may also be physiologic (a normal occurrence in the body), as when new blood vessels sprout in response to the chronic state of low oxygen that characterizes the inadequate flow of blood in heart disease. When the heart receives insufficient oxygen, this signals the body to build more blood vessels, called collaterals.

Angiogenesis has shown promise in the treatment of *ischemic* heart disease, which is heart disease caused by inadequate blood flow. The building of these collateral blood vessels can be facilitated by gene therapy, in which genes controlling angiogenesis are injected directly onto the surface of the heart. These genes then promote the development of new pathways through which blood can travel to nourish the heart muscle.

Exciting research is focusing on the use of gene therapy to treat coronary artery disease. Clinical trials are aimed at assessing its effectiveness in heart patients who have no other treatment options. Perhaps, in the future, bypass surgery will become obsolete, replaced by a simple injection of genes to treat coronary artery disease.

Jim peered out the window and grunted at the heavy snowfall. It was December, and a white Christmas was expected, but on this Sunday morning his two teenagers wouldn't be out of bed for at least another three hours. He reluctantly put on his old boots, zipped his coat over his generous girth and rummaged through the glove box before spearing a pair of gloves and a toque. When he stepped outside, he found himself in heavy wet snow that came up to his knees.

Jim was fifty-three. He was overweight, out of shape and sedentary. Ten years ago he had quit smoking. Although his blood pressure and cholesterol were elevated, he had spent the last few years fending off the medications recommended by his physician; Jim worried about side effects, and his doctor could not assure him that the drugs were completely safe.

Jim's breath heaved with each shovelful of snow, and it took him twenty minutes to clear half the driveway. He was sweaty and his heart was pounding in his chest. As he lifted another shovel load he felt a fist crush his chest. He dropped the shovel and staggered up the driveway, grasping the side of the garage to keep his balance. Weak from the pain, he inched his way inside and croaked out his wife's name. He vomited and the pain intensified.

"Call an ambulance," he whispered to his startled wife. "I think I'm having a heart attack."

The paramedics found Jim pale and sweaty, clutching his chest and sitting in the kitchen. They rapidly inserted an intravenous line into his forearm, administered oxygen by nasal prongs and loaded him into the ambulance. Lights flashing and siren blaring, the ambulance reached the hospital in eight minutes and deposited Jim in the acute area of the emergency room.

The triage nurse took one look at Jim and summoned the emergency room physician. Jim's blood pressure was low, his heart rate high. He was short of breath, pale and perspiring heavily. Staff members swarmed his gurney, quickly removing his snow shoveling gear.

After scanning the electrocardiogram, the emergency room doctor told the charge nurse, "This one is massive. See if the cardiologist on call is still in the hospital." The attending cardiologist rushed down to emergency, and after assessing the ECG and examining Jim he summoned the angioplasty team.

Jim's left anterior descending coronary artery was blocked.

But he was lucky. Not only was he transported to the hospital quickly, but angioplasty facilities were available on site. He received the best available care. The blocked artery was opened with angioplasty and a stent was deployed to keep it open.

Afterward, Jim was left with only mild heart weakness. He was admonished to take his risk factors more seriously, and a diet and exercise program was set up. It was also made very clear to him that, while his fear of drug side effects was not uncommon, this risk was far outweighed by the dangers he faced if he didn't treat his heart problem. Jim was discharged from hospital five days after admission, on a cocktail of cardiac medications. When he got home, he informed his kids that in future *they* would clean the driveway after snowfalls.

5. Angioplasty and Bypass Surgery

The treatment of coronary artery disease may be invasive or non-invasive (also known as medical). Every heart patient is treated medically. This includes lifestyle modification and drugs to lower cholesterol, reduce angina, lower blood pressure, etc. An invasive approach, involving coronary artery angioplasty (*percutaneous transluminal coronary angioplasty,* or *PTCA*) or coronary bypass surgery is neither suitable nor indicated for every patient with CAD.

Some patients with stable angina and low-risk stress and perfusion tests may not require an invasive approach. The risk of intervening, though small, may be equal to or greater than the risk of a heart attack. Other patients may not be interventional candidates for the opposite reason. Even though they experience severe angina and have high-risk CAD, their coronary arteries may be too small and diffusely diseased to repair with either angioplasty or surgery. As with all medical procedures, the decision to undertake coronary artery angioplasty and coronary artery bypass surgery should be made after a careful evaluation of risks and benefits.

Coronary Angiograms

A coronary angiogram is the gold standard in the diagnosis of coronary artery disease. It is the best test for determining the presence of CAD and the degree of narrowing.

Coronary angiogram

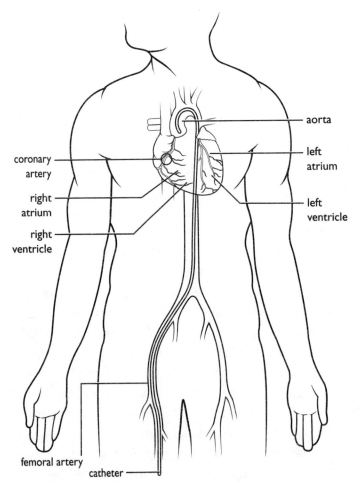

The results of common diagnostic procedures such as electrocardiograms, stress tests and perfusion tests, combined with a history and physical exam, determine whether you need a coronary angiogram. During an angiogram, a thin hollow catheter (tube) is placed into a blood vessel (the femoral artery) in the leg. The catheter is guided up the artery into the aorta and positioned just above the heart. Dye is then injected through the tube and into the coronary arteries, and X-rays are taken. If any coronary arteries have become too narrow to let enough blood through, the angiogram will show the bottleneck.

Risks of Coronary Angiography

Why isn't an angiogram offered to everyone with chest pain? Why bother with stress tests and perfusion studies? It's because coronary angiograms are invasive tests, and are therefore associated with risk. (Everything in medicine boils down to risk.) Threading the catheter up the aorta into the mouths of the coronary arteries (each opening is called an *ostium*) is potentially dangerous. Complications can include possibly fatal heart attacks, strokes, kidney damage and arterial bleeding at the site of entry in the leg. Unfortunately, a doctor can't accurately predict who will suffer a complication, any more than a police officer can predict which car will be involved in an accident. On the other hand, just as a car with worn tires is at greater risk of an accident, some people are at greater risk of developing complications from coronary angiography. The risk depends on your age and heart function, and the presence of other illnesses, such as diabetes. The older and sicker you are, the greater the perils of testing. The risk also depends on the severity of the coronary artery disease. People with very severe CAD have a 1 in 100 to 1 in 200 chance of dying during the procedure.

The likelihood of death is considerably higher if the disease goes undetected. Death rates are only one important variable in the treatment decision. In addition to mortality (risk of death), *morbidity* must also be considered. Morbidity is the chance that the procedure (or the lack of the procedure) may lead to something that seriously interferes with your enjoyment of life. This may include a stroke, heart attack or kidney failure.

Because of the risks, an angiogram is not done routinely, like an ECG or stress test. Most people with chest pain do not have coronary artery disease, and routine angiograms would expose them to unnecessary and unacceptable danger. In addition, because angiograms are expensive, routine testing would be too costly.

Randomized studies

When you have a heart condition and surgery is proposed, there's an obvious question: what are the chances of survival if the condition is ignored, compared to the chances of survival with surgery? The most reliable predictions come from randomized studies. In a randomized study, once someone agrees to participate and accept the therapy offered by the trial, an envelope is randomly selected. It contains one of two (or more) treatments. For example, in a study of left main coronary artery disease, the envelope mandates either medications or surgery. The study continues for a predetermined amount of time, and during that time records are fastidiously checked to see how the participants in each group are faring. At the end of the study period (whether it is fifty years, five years, five days or five minutes), the data are collected and the results are reported. In the case of left main coronary artery disease, studies proved that the risk of dying within five years was 80 percent on medication and only 25 percent with surgery.

Patients who might otherwise have survived may die from surgical complications. There may also be patients who are alive after five years on medication who would have died during surgery. But, barring these exceptions, which group would you prefer to join—the one with twenty individuals dead at the end of five years, or the group with seventy-five?

The Angiogram

Most people scheduled for angiograms arrive at the hospital on the day of the procedure. Barring complications, or severe CAD requiring urgent therapy, they go home later that same day. Although the procedure resembles an operation, with masked, green-robed staff rushing about, it is only a diagnostic test. Patients wear a standard issue hospital gown and are required to lie on a narrow, stone-cold steel table.

The test itself is surprisingly smooth and painless. It is commonly performed through the femoral artery, at the groin area. More recent techniques allow for access through the radial artery (at the wrist) in some people, but while this is preferable, it is not always possible to gain access to the radial artery.

You remain conscious during the angiogram. First, a needle is used to inject local anesthetic, to freeze the area and minimize your discomfort. Then the angiogram catheter is inserted. The insides of the arteries and the heart don't feel the catheter, and there should be no discomfort until it is removed at the end of the test.

Dye is injected into the mouths of your coronary arteries and flows down the length of the blood vessels. A large camera rotates around your body, taking two-dimensional pictures of the blood vessels, now filled with dye. Any narrowing along the length of an artery will quickly become apparent.

At the end of the procedure, the catheter may be maneuvered into the left ventricle of your heart. A larger volume of dye is then injected to make the whole chamber opaque. (You get a feeling like the warm flush that follows a shot of whiskey.) This part of the test is called a *ventriculogram*, and it assesses heart function. In the era of echocardiograms, the ventriculogram is nearly obsolete, except in rare circumstances. Inexplicably, it continues to be performed routinely.

The next stage of the procedure involves pulling the catheter out of the femoral artery. This can cause bleeding, so pressure is applied manually, and then a clamp is placed over the artery for fifteen to thirty minutes, followed by the application of a small sandbag. While the clamp is being applied, the results are relayed to you and any family at your bedside. For the next four hours you will be required to lie flat, without bending your legs or raising your head.

Most of the complaints about angiograms center around the post-angiogram period. People don't like to lie motionless for hours. Bruising of the groin and thigh is common. Occasionally small (and sometimes large) blood clots, called *hematomas*, form. Very rarely, surgery is needed to repair a damaged femoral artery.

Angioplasty and Stents

"Angio" means "blood vessel" and "plasty" means "to fix." Once an important narrowing of the artery (stenosis) has been identified, the dilemma is how to fix it and reduce the chance of a heart attack. Is the narrowing best dealt with by angioplasty or bypass surgery? In the 1960s and 1970s, the standard treatment for most heart disease was coronary bypass—a major operation involving splitting the sternum (breastbone) and cutting into the heart. The introduction of coronary angioplasty was revolutionary. This procedure, which is performed in the same way as coronary angiography, represented a much less invasive alternative for fixing blood vessels.

Coronary angioplasty was first performed in Zurich, in 1977, by a German physician named Andreas Gruentzig. His first patient, a thirty-eight-year-old smoker named Adolph Bachman, is still alive (he has quit smoking). Gruentzig first toyed with catheters in his kitchen, and in 1976 he presented animal data to a skeptical group. Today, in the United States, more than 700,000 angioplasties are carried out per year; in Canada the figure is 12,000 to 13,000. While working in

Atlanta in 1985, Gruentzig piloted a private plane to his death during a storm.

Nearly all patients would prefer angioplasty to bypass surgery. No one wants a split-open chest and several weeks of recuperation when angioplasty allows discharge from hospital the same day, with rapid resumption of activities. However, angioplasty is not always feasible. Lengthy narrowings, and narrowings around the curve of an artery, may be too technically difficult for angioplasty, so bypass surgery is sometimes required.

Angioplasty and a stent

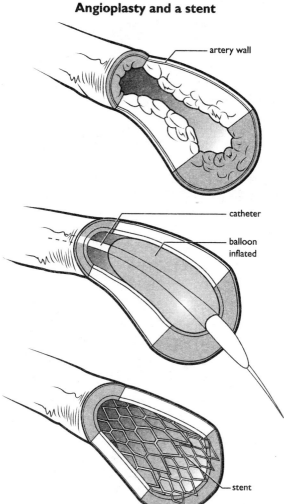

artery wall

catheter

balloon inflated

stent

Drug-eluting stents (DES)

Drug-eluting stents are the latest major breakthrough in interventional cardiology. The outer wall of a drug-eluting stent is coated with a thin polymer of a drug, slowly released into the arterial tissue. The drug acts to inhibit growth of inflammatory cells involved in the process of re-stenosis. The drugs used include rapamycin, an antibiotic and potent immunosuppressive agent used to prevent organ transplant rejection, and pactitaxel, a chemotherapeutic agent and anti-metabolite.

Drug-eluting stents are now available throughout the world, and have been shown to significantly reduce the rate of re-stenosis. As with most new technologies, however, the cost of each stent is very high. Therefore, the use of DES is likely to be initially restricted to those arteries at the highest risk of re-stenosis, and those patients who can afford to pay.

The Mechanics of Angioplasty

Angioplasty involves placing a very small wire across the narrowing (lesion) in the artery. A small hot-dog-shaped balloon is then positioned over the wire, within the narrowing, and is inflated with liquid to squish the fat in the arterial walls, opening up the artery. There are a series of these balloon inflations, each lasting under a minute. This is similar to what happens during a heart attack, as no blood can flow through the artery during the inflation. Fortunately, blocking the flow for such brief periods rarely has adverse consequences, and causes no significant heart damage.

During one such procedure, many narrowings can be angioplastied. However, each procedure increases the likelihood that at least one blood vessel will become narrowed again in the future. This unfortunate complication occurs in about 10 percent of patients within six months of the procedure. The risk of renarrowing can be reduced by inserting a cylindrical wire mesh tube (a *stent*) into the angioplastied area. This procedure was first performed in France in 1986. A stent can only be positioned after the vessel has been widened by angioplasty. Each of the more than twenty stents available in North

America costs thousands of dollars. Some people end up with five, six or even more stents, but most require only one or two. After successful angioplasty and stenting, expensive blood thinners are used to reduce the risk of sudden renarrowing.

Risks of Angioplasty

The risks of angioplasty are similar to those of angiography, although slightly higher. The death rate is greater, at 1 in 500. Minor heart attacks can occur during the procedure. There is a 1 percent chance that the patient will require emergency bypass surgery due to technical failure, such as abrupt closure of an artery, either during the angioplasty or thereafter. The chance of a blood vessel suddenly closing is 1 in 200. Thus, angioplasty should only be performed in centers with cardiac surgical backup, where the patient can be whisked into the operating room. If the angioplasty fails and there is no surgery available on site, the results can be catastrophic.

Jack tapped his foot as he stood in the corridor, waiting for the angiography office to open. It was seven in the morning and he was going to have to wait another thirty minutes. He had awakened at five a.m. after a fitful sleep, so he and his wife, Ruth, had driven to the hospital early. Now Ruth stood by his side, clasping his hand. She was stoic, as usual, but after forty-two years of marriage he knew she was as nervous as he.

Jack had suffered five months of increasingly frequent angina, punctuated by treadmill tests and new medications. Now came the most invasive test, a coronary angiogram. Jack's cardiologist had explained that the angiogram was the only way to identify the presence and extent of coronary artery disease. At first Jack had declined, concerned about the small risk of stroke and heart attack. But within a week, Ruth and his children had changed his mind. Now, resigned to the need for the test, Jack feared the results.

Finally the receptionist arrived and directed Jack to a room where he could don a hospital gown. The nurse informed Jack that he was fourth on the list, and that she anticipated that he'd be wheeled into the angiogram room just before lunch. The hours rolled by slowly. By two in the afternoon, Jack's anxiety was mixed with equal parts of annoyance. His kids had already arrived, assuming that the procedure would be over by then.

Thirty minutes later, two nurses loaded Jack onto the stretcher, and he waved to his family as he rolled down the hall to the cath lab. The cardiologist was in surgical greens and masked. Jack transferred himself to the steel cath lab table, shimmying across from the gurney. His groin was shaved and prepped with sterile solution. With a few seconds of warning, a small needle penetrated the skin over his left groin and raised a small bleb (a collection of blood under the skin). The local freezing rapidly took effect. A plastic catheter was inserted into his femoral artery and threaded up to his heart. Jack couldn't feel the catheter, since the insides of blood vessels don't sense pain. A large camera circled his head, taking pictures as the dye was injected up into his coronary arteries. He heard the medical staff discussing the results, but he couldn't understand the conversation that shot across the room. Within fifteen minutes of his arrival, the test was complete and the cardiologist was explaining his results.

"It looks like a single vessel is affected." the doctor told Jack. "I think we should be able to angioplasty it, but we can't do it today. I'll come by your room in ten minutes and remove the sheath from your groin. I can talk to you and your family about the options then."

It turned out that Jack was lucky. Only one vessel was affected, and he wouldn't need bypass surgery. When a single coronary artery is narrowed, it is typically repaired with angioplasty; bypass surgery is rarely required in these cases. Jack had successful angioplasty the following week, and he and Ruth were far less nervous the second time around, because the angioplasty procedure was so similar to the angiogram.

Coronary Artery Bypass Grafting (CABG)

Bypass surgery is performed by cardiac surgeons. The technical expertise of heart surgery often goes unrecognized by patients and their families. Cardiovascular surgeons routinely perform miracles. Their physical skills are matched by superior mental stamina and concentration. They deserve seven-figure signing bonuses and yearly salaries to match.

Experimental bypass surgery was begun by an Argentinian doctor named Rene Favaloro, who died in 2000 of a self-inflicted gunshot wound. Bypass was first performed on humans in 1962 by Dr. David Sabiston at Johns Hopkins Medical Center in Baltimore. The surgery is called bypass for two reasons. The coronary narrowing is "bypassed" by diverting the blood flow to another blood vessel. As well, heart and lungs are "bypassed" and temporarily replaced by a machine, to allow the surgeon to operate on a cold, immobile heart, since complex surgery would be impossible on a heart that was quivering and pumping.

Coronary artery bypass grafting (CABG, pronounced cabbage) is Russian in origin, with animal models first reported by Dr. Vasilly Ivanovich Kolessov. It is a revolutionary procedure that uses the patient's own artery or vein. At the start of surgery, the blood vessel for the bypass is removed. One end is stitched to the aorta and the other end is attached to the coronary artery just beyond the narrowing. Veins are removed from the patient's legs, and arteries can be taken from a number of different areas, including the chest and arm. For example, everyone has a left and right internal mammary artery (LIMA and RIMA), which arise from the aorta and supply blood to the chest wall. Because the chest is also supplied by other arteries, the RIMA and LIMA are redundant and can be used as conduits for bypass. They are dissected out of the chest, and the bottom end is cut and reattached to the coronary artery.

Coronary artery bypass graft

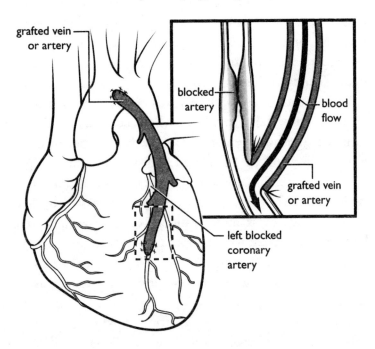

grafted vein
or artery

blocked
artery

blood
flow

grafted vein
or artery

left blocked
coronary
artery

Another artery commonly used in bypass surgery is the radial artery, which runs the length of the forearm and supplies blood to the hand. Luckily, most people have a dual blood supply to the hand. If the radial artery is removed, the ulnar artery provides more than enough blood.

Arteries are more reliable conduits than veins. The likelihood of an artery remaining open ten years after bypass is about 90 percent. The likelihood of a vein remaining open at ten years is about 50 percent. Surgeons therefore try to use arteries for bypass whenever possible. Why use veins at all? Unfortunately, many people require multiple bypasses, and there simply aren't enough arteries available. Also, using arteries for bypass takes longer, and the longer the operation, the greater the risk of complications. Accordingly, to reduce operation time, emergency bypasses are typically done using veins.

Choosing the Treatment

Before a treatment decision is made, an angiogram is used to supply details of the coronary anatomy. Depending on the case, interventions like angioplasty or bypass surgery may not be technically possible. Even for someone who has severe symptoms, there may be nothing to offer but medication to control the symptoms and reduce the risk of hospitalization. In other cases, although a narrowing may be technically reparable, it may not be necessary to fix it. Perhaps the blood vessel is only moderately narrowed, or the person has minimal symptoms.

If the coronary arteries should be fixed, and can be fixed, many factors determine how the abnormal arteries should be repaired. These factors include the number of narrowed arteries, the site of disease, other medical conditions (the person may be too sick to undergo bypass surgery) and the person's

The limits of bypass

There are limitations to the cardiovascular surgeon's ability. If the entire blood vessel is littered with narrowings, there is no way to bypass them all; not only would it take too much time, and therefore be too dangerous, but it would be technically impossible. Likewise, if the portion of the artery beyond the narrowing is too small to allow attachment of another blood vessel, bypass is ruled out. No matter how skilled the surgeon, a normal-sized blood vessel cannot be stitched into an artery the width of a hair; even microsurgery would permit only a few drops of blood to pass through, which would be useless. Finally, if the narrowing occurs at the end of the blood vessel (a condition known as *distal disease*) bypass is much less useful.

wishes. Even if statistics point to bypass surgery as the superior choice, this does not mean that angioplasty is contraindi-
cated. Some people prefer to take their chances, and opt for
angioplasty, as it is much less invasive than splitting the sternum.

While it can be difficult to determine whether angioplasty
or bypass is the better option, in some cases the choice is clear.
For example, when the left main coronary artery is narrowed,
the sole option is bypass. The left main is akin to a tree trunk;
it's the origin of the entire left coronary system. Drug treatment
of left main disease carries an extremely high mortality rate of
30 percent by eighteen months. Angioplasty is ruled out because
there is a high risk that the inflated balloon will cut off blood
flow to the left side of the heart, resulting in cardiac arrest. Similarly, triple vessel disease, in which all three major blood vessels
are narrowed, is a problem best solved with bypass surgery.
However, techniques of angioplasty and bypass are continually
being refined, with new treatment options altering what was
once held as dogma. In these shifting seas, the best options for
coronary disease may quickly change.

When planning bypass surgery, the doctor must assess the
left ventricular function, or LVF, of your heart. LVF is the most
important factor in the prognosis after a heart attack. The
portion of heart muscle that dies in a heart attack becomes scar
tissue, and can no more recover its function than a hand can
regrow a lost finger. If the blocked blood vessel supplies only
a small amount of heart muscle, cardiac function will be only
mildly affected. But if the artery supplies a large amount of
muscle, the ramifications are desperate. When more than 40
percent of the muscle is destroyed (infarcted), the heart is too
weak to supply the body with sufficient blood for normal functions and the body goes into cardiogenic shock, with a mortality rate of more than 90 percent. In very small heart attacks,
mortality rates may be as low as 2 percent.

Cardiovascular surgery is a prime example of the vast distance medicine has traversed in mere decades. Our ability to mend broken hearts, and deliver years of quality life to people who not long ago would have died prematurely, is a stunning feat of innovation, ingenuity and skill.

Heart Transplants

The first transplant of a human heart was performed on December 3, 1967, in Groote Schuur Hospital, Cape Town, South Africa, on a fifty-four-year-old Lithuanian-born grocer named Louis Washkansky. The pioneering operation was performed by Dr. Christiaan Barnard. The heart was donated by the family of twenty-three-year-old Denise Durvall, who had been hit by a car. Though the transplant was categorized as successful, Mr. Washkansky died of pneumonia eighteen days later. The second recipient of a successful heart transplant, Philip Blaiberg, lived for nineteen months after surgery. In between these two operations, an American team in New York failed when the transplant recipient died after six hours.

These days, some 150 to 175 heart transplantations are performed each year in Canada. In the United States there are 2,000 to 2,500 heart transplants per year. The two-year survival rate is 85 percent and the five-year survival rate is 70 percent.

Heart transplants remain the last resort for individuals with severe heart failure. Only patients with a life expectancy below twelve months are considered potential candidates. In order to combat organ rejection—one of the most serious complications of transplant surgery—the recipient will have to take a complex cocktail of anti-rejection medications for the rest of his or her life. Side effects of these vital drugs include a higher incidence of infections and accelerated blood vessel narrowing (atherosclerosis). As well, the incidence of various forms of cancer, including skin cancer, is raised more than a hundredfold in people who have had heart transplants. In effect, heart transplantation exchanges one disease for others. The benefit, of course, is the many years a heart transplant can add to someone's life.

Transplantation programs are associated with fame and profits. As a result, transplant centers have sprung up like donut shops in many areas of the United States. So far, this has not happened in Canada, due to tighter government control of health care.

Studies have shown that the best long-term results are achieved in hospitals that perform the greatest number of transplants. Therefore, surgery at a center that conducts only five operations a year is far less desirable than surgery at a center that conducts fifty a year. But desperate patients and their families take what they can get. If a shack in rural Arkansas were the only hospital offering the surgery, most people with six months to live would jump at the chance.

6. Arrhythmias

Normally, the heart beats regularly, rhythmically and soothingly. We are oblivious of its rate and rhythm as the heart silently ensures we are at the correct "speed" during our daily activities.

Normal rhythm is called *sinus rhythm*. The sinus node (also called the *sino-atrial* or *SA node*) is the heart's electrical generator. It is a very small structure composed of a tangle of specialized cells embedded in the atrium. The sinus node receives signals from the brain and body instructing it to increase or decrease the heart rate according to need. The signal moves from the node through the atrium to the *atrioventricular node (AV node)*, another tangle of special cells, which functions as a gatekeeper or checkpoint on the electrical road. The AV node receives the signal and sends it forward to the main pumping chambers (the ventricles). However, the heart has an interesting protective mechanism in case the heart rate becomes too rapid. If the AV node is bombarded with signals, it will delay the signals at its checkpoint, a function called *decremental conduction*. This action prevents the heart rate from reaching a speed that would endanger life. Most people cannot increase their heart rate beyond 190 to 200 beats per minute.

The heart's electrical system can malfunction in a number of ways. It can do so independently, or in relation to another

Arrhythmias

"Arrhythmia" is a catchall word meaning a problem in the heart's electrical system. It may refer to a single skipped beat, which everyone experiences at times, or to a life-threatening rapid pulse requiring emergency medical attention. It does not define the nature of the problem, or its seriousness.

heart ailment. Electrophysiology (EP) is a separate cardiology specialty that deals specifically with these electrical malfunctions. Over the past twenty years, EP research into the workings and foibles of the cardiac electrical system has multiplied.

Tachycardia

Tachycardia is defined as a rapid heart rate ("tachy" comes from the Greek word for "fast"). Any heart rate above 100 beats per minute is a tachycardia, even if it is an appropriate response to the circumstances. For example, a sinus tachycardia is expected when activities are sufficiently strenuous. Exercise is supposed to raise the heart rate; an inability to increase the heart rate during exercise may be a sign of serious disease.

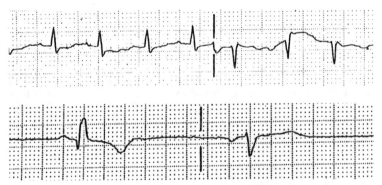

Above, a section of an ECG showing tachycardia. Each spike represents a heartbeat, and the heart rate is 133 beats per minute. Below, an ECG showing bradycardia, with a heart rate of 38 beats per minute.

Bradycardia

Bradycardia refers to a slow heart rate, defined as under 50 beats per minute. (*Bradus* is Greek for "slow.") A physically fit person has a lower than average resting heart rate because exercise creates a more efficient heart and body. Whereas the resting heart rate is lower in a fit person, the maximum heart rate with exercise is the same, but an unfit individual who exercises reaches a fast heart rate sooner than an athlete does.

It has been suggested that the average resting heart rate in mammals is inversely proportional to life span. Small rodents, for example, have heart rates of 300 beats per minute, and live only a few years.

There is no normal heart rate, but there is a normal range. Most people have resting heart rates of 60 to 85 beats per minute, but rates under 60 are often normal. Rates under 50 are less often normal, and rates under 40 are never normal. As the electrical system ages, the heart rate naturally slows down. It is common for elderly people to develop low heart rates.

Bradycardia can be due to cardiac medications—specifically beta-blockers, some calcium-channel blockers and anti-arrhythmic drugs, including amiodarone, propafenone, procainamide, quinidine and flecainide (see Chapter 10). Often, bradycardia is not a side effect but is the expected and even intended effect of a cardiac medication. However, excessive bradycardia can develop unexpectedly as a result of these drugs, in which case either the dose should be reduced or the drug should be discontinued. For that reason, it's wise to start these medications at a low dose and increase them gradually, under careful supervision, to either prevent developing an excessively low heart rate, or identify the side effect quickly.

Bradycardia is also an important complication of many cardiac conditions. The more slowly the heart beats, the less oxygen it uses. In a person with impaired blood flow because of coronary artery disease, a slow heartbeat may be desirable. Some heart attacks, especially those involving blockage of the right coronary artery (RCA), are associated with inappropriately low heart rates. The RCA supplies blood to much of the heart's electrical system, so when it is blocked the electrical system can be damaged. Any severe cardiac condition may be complicated by bradycardia. If the doors, walls or plumbing of a house are damaged, the electrical system is likely to be affected also.

Symptoms of bradycardia range from fatigue to loss of consciousness. If the bradycardia develops insidiously and you are inactive, you may feel little more than fatigue and shortness of breath with exertion. If your heart rate continues to slow, you may develop lightheadedness. If your heart rate continues to slow down you may lose consciousness (a condition called *syncope*) because your blood pressure will be too low to support normal brain activity. Symptoms depend on how low the heart rate dives. A heart rate of 40 is less likely to cause syncope than a heart rate of 20.

People who have become unconscious often find themselves in a hospital emergency room. If the problem was caused by transient bradycardia, it may not be apparent to the doctor; the heart rate may be normal in the emergency department, and the person may be discharged without a diagnosis. However, some people arrive at the hospital with obvious bradycardia and hypotension (low blood pressure) and receive the emergency therapy they require.

Pacemakers

Pacemaker technology was developed in 1930 by New York City cardiologist Dr. Albert Hyman. The device was first implanted in a patient in 1958, in Sweden, by Ake Senning, a surgeon, and Rune Elmqvist, an engineer. The patient was forty-three-year-old Arn Larsson, who was suffering from life-threatening bradycardia. Mr. Larsson had multiple surgical adjustments during his life, including twenty-two different pacemakers. He died of cancer on December 28, 2001, having had his life span doubled by the devices.

A pacemaker is a backup system that monitors the electrical activity of the heart and responds to a slow heart rate by zapping the heart into action. Think of it as a warden with a whip, overseeing a prisoner breaking rocks in the quarry. Every time the prisoner fails to swing the pick, the whip cracks down. Modern pacemakers are small, and weigh as little as half an ounce (15 g). The pacemaker includes a titanium pulse generator that contains both computer circuitry and the battery. The pulse generator, which is slightly larger than a matchbox, is surgically implanted under the skin and muscles of the left chest, just below the collarbone. The surgery is minor (unless you are the one under the scalpel), taking no more than an hour or two. Patients are lightly sedated to take the edge off the discomfort, and the procedure is completed under local anesthetic. One or two long insulated wires (leads) are connected to the pulse generator, and travel from there through a vein to the heart, and into the right atrium and/or ventricle.

Pacemakers are either single-chamber or dual-chamber devices. In a single-chamber pacer, one lead attaches to either the right atrium or, more commonly, the right ventricle. In a dual-chamber device there are two leads, one in the right atrium and the other in the right ventricle.

Pacemakers are smart devices. The lead monitors the heart's electrical activity, sending a report to the pulse generator with each beat. If too much time elapses between heartbeats (bradycardia), the pulse generator transmits an electrical signal down the length of the wire into the heart muscle, triggering a heartbeat. If the cardiologist has programmed the pacemaker for a heart rate of 60, it will activate a heartbeat only if one full second elapses without an intrinsic beat. If the pacemaker has been set to a low rate of 50, slightly more than one second must elapse without a heartbeat before the pacemaker kicks in.

A dual-chambered pacemaker

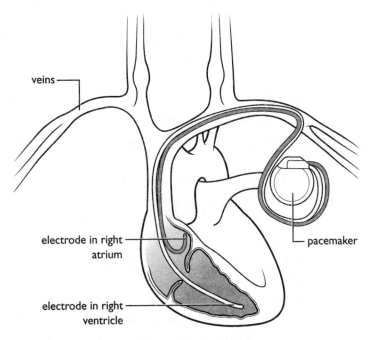

The battery life of a pacemaker depends upon how often it is being used, as not all people with bradycardia suffer from the condition twenty-four hours a day. The range is about eight to fifteen years. When the battery runs out (this is closely monitored by a cardiologist and anticipated months in advance), it can be replaced in a simple outpatient procedure.

Most people can be discharged the day following implantation. There may be routine bruising around the implantation site. Collections of blood (hematomas) around the site are less common, but do occur; people taking the blood-thinner warfarin are particularly prone to minor bleeding. Infection is very rare.

There is no need to curtail your activities after a pacemaker is inserted. Sexual activity may resume. Since a pacer is an electrical appliance, its function can be affected by close proximity to some electrical devices such as power lines, but only if you climb them. Radiation can also influence pacemaker function; however, it's prudent to avoid radiation even if you don't have a pacemaker. Cellphones may briefly interfere with pacemaker function, but the risk has been overstated. As a precaution, don't wear a cellphone in a pocket directly over the pacer.

There are many different types of bradycardia. Some of them require a pacemaker even if you don't have symptoms, while others should only be treated with this device if you have significant lightheadedness or loss of consciousness. In an emergency, a temporary pacemaker may be inserted either at the bedside or under fluoroscopy (X-ray guidance) in an angiogram laboratory.

Pacemakers are safe and easy to insert, and they have the potential to dramatically improve the quality of life for people with symptomatic bradycardia.

Skipped Beats

Everyone experiences occasional premature contractions, otherwise known as skipped (or extra) heartbeats, but they are a source of enormous anxiety for many people. While any form of heart disease can be associated with skipped beats, most people with skipped beats do not have a heart problem.

When a skipped beat arises in an atrium, it's called a premature atrial beat, or atrial ectopic beat. When one is initiated in a ventricle, it is termed a premature ventricular beat, or premature ventricular contraction.

In most cases, skipped beats are only as important as the symptoms they cause. As a general rule they are irrelevant to cardiac health, with no relationship to heart disease and no impact on life span.

However, if you do have a heart disease you are much more likely to experience skipped beats, due to the irritability of a diseased heart muscle. After a heart attack, the number of extra beats is inversely proportional to the chance of survival: the more extra beats, the higher the mortality rate. This finding led to a study (called the CAST trial) that used a drug to inhibit the number of skipped beats. It was assumed that if the extra beats were reduced, mortality would improve. The trial was terminated early. Although the drug was reducing the extra beats, people taking the drug were more likely to die than those taking a placebo. The CAST trial is an example of why therapies need to be tested before they are widely used.

The list of causes for skipped beats is long, and includes alcohol, drugs, caffeine, aging, lack of sleep and many other conditions. However, just because your heart skips beats, you do not necessarily require tests to search for an associated condition. It should be obvious from a history and physical exam whether anything untoward is going on. In an otherwise well person, a normal cardiac ultrasound and stress test should be enough to allay fears of impending death.

Occasionally, symptoms of extra beats are so troubling that treatment is required. The usual choice is a beta-blocker. The dilemma, as always, is that you trade your symptoms for the potential side effects of the medication. But if palpitations are incapacitating for you, initiating a beta-blocker and evaluating the results is a reasonable choice.

Atrial Fibrillation

Atrial fibrillation (*a.fib*) is an arrhythmia that is common, annoying and difficult to treat. What is this frustrating heart problem?

The sinus node is an electrical workhorse, and any heart disease can interfere with its proper function. When the sinus node is damaged, instead of producing an orderly progression of heartbeats, the atrium can become hyperactive. When this occurs, the AV node is bombarded with up to 600 electrical impulses per minute. If your heart were to beat at a rate of 400 to 600 times a minute, it (and you) would turn into a quivering mass of jelly. The AV node works as a gatekeeper to allow only a portion of the excessive impulses to cross over and generate a heartbeat. Unfortunately, the node often becomes overwhelmed and allows too many through. The result is a disorganized, irregular and rapid heartbeat, often between 130 and 170 beats per minute.

The irregularity of the beats is secondary to the massive influx of signals. If a bouncer is trying to prevent patrons from getting through a door and he becomes overwhelmed, people will not rush forward in an orderly manner. Like the atrial fibrillation signals, they will plow through in fits and starts. This inefficiency cannot be sustained for long. A.fib causes palpitations, shortness of breath and chest pain, and is usually so uncomfortable when it begins that people find themselves banging at the emergency room door. Rapid atrial fibrillation is usually serious enough to warrant admission to an emergency room bed.

Atrial fibrillation may be associated with any type of heart disease. It is particularly common if you have hypertension, heart attacks, congestive heart failure or valve disease. It may also occur after alcohol binges and with thyroid disease. About 10 percent of the time, especially in younger people, no cause or association can be identified; this is referred to as *lone atrial fibrillation*.

Treatment

Not all people with atrial fibrillation have the same symptoms. Some are already taking rate slowing drugs, or have aged electrical systems. Although still irregular, their heart rate may be less than 100. Some appear in the doctor's office feeling "off" but not unwell enough to be hospitalized. Others may appear shockingly asymptomatic despite a rapidly beating heart but will become sick if their a.fib goes untreated. Most are "tachying" along too quickly and need to be slowed down.

The first step in managing atrial fibrillation is controlling the heart rate. One of the most predictable ways to slow down the heart is with intravenous or oral beta-blockers; these are excellent rate-slowing drugs. A more expensive alternative is calcium-channel blockers. Digoxin is commonly used to slow the heart rate but is becoming obsolete with the development of newer and more effective medication. Digoxin is ineffective for reducing the frequency of atrial fibrillation; people taking it are just as likely to develop recurrent atrial fibrillation as those without it. Additionally, digoxin is much less effective in reducing the heart rate during atrial fibrillation than either beta-blockers or calcium-channel blockers. Because digoxin is excreted by the kidneys, if there is any change in kidney function (which is often unrecognized by patients), there is a danger of developing digoxin toxicity.

After the heart rate is controlled, it may be converted back into normal sinus rhythm. The drugs that control heart rate (beta-blockers and some calcium-channel blockers) cannot achieve this goal. Other drugs used to treat many arrhythmias are appropriately called anti-arrhythmics, and not only slow down a rapid heart rate but also effectively transform atrial fibrillation into a normal rhythm. Examples of anti-arrhythmics include sotalol, amiodarone, propafenone and flecainide. For more details on these medications, see Chapter 10.

The dilemma is that these drugs are not always effective (not many drugs are always effective), and they may have side effects. If one drug is ineffective, a second or third can be tried.

About 50 percent of people who have paroxysms of atrial fibrillation will have further attacks despite taking either propafenone or sotalol. Amiodarone is the most effective drug, with a recurrence rate of about 30 percent within two years. Unfortunately, amiodarone has more side effects than propafenone or sotalol.

The decision to use anti-arrhythmics is complex. If you are very symptomatic from atrial fibrillation, anti-arrhythmic therapy may be necessary. Yet some people have almost no symptoms despite being in atrial fibrillation all the time. In these cases, a safer "rate-controlling" drug may suffice.

Atrial Fibrillation and Strokes

Why should you even consider using drugs for atrial fibrillation if you don't have symptoms? Because atrial fibrillation can cause strokes. As the atria fibrillate, the blood in the chambers swirls as aimlessly as a rudderless ship until it crosses over into the ventricles. In this environment, atrial clots are more likely to form. Clots do not necessarily stick to the ventricle walls; they may be catapulted out of the heart and into the brain. If this catastrophe occurs, the clot is propelled through smaller and smaller arteries within the brain until it blocks one, causing a stroke—a cerebrovascular accident (CVA). As in a heart attack, when blood flow is blocked, the area supplied by the blocked artery dies.

The risk of stroke being caused by atrial fibrillation is increased by hypertension, diabetes, a history of a previous stroke, certain types of valve disease, age over sixty-five and heart failure. The more risk factors someone has, the more likely it is that a stroke will occur. For a person with no risks, the chance of a stroke is low. While the likelihood of a stroke is quoted at about 4 percent per year, the percentage can be much higher in patients with multiple risks. The good news is that stroke risk can be sharply reduced to 1.5 percent per year with the daily use of warfarin (referred to by some as rat poison).

Warfarin thins the blood, inhibiting clots by inhibiting the action of vitamin K. Vitamin K is an important element in the liver's manufacture of certain proteins in the blood called clotting factors. If these factors are not synthesized by the liver, blood clotting takes longer. Aspirin is also a blood thinner, but much weaker.

When used in atrial fibrillation, warfarin reduces clot formation within the atria, thereby reducing the risk of stroke. For every thirty people with atrial fibrillation who take warfarin, one stroke is prevented each year, although it does cause one or two serious bleeding episodes per thousand patients per year. Strokes are a common and greatly feared possibility for heart patients. They can result in loss of mobility, speech and independence.

Unfortunately, many people find taking warfarin to be a nuisance, since it only works effectively if it is taken according to a strict dosing regimen that requires rigid compliance. The regimen is different for each patient. Since your blood must not be too thick or too thin, you will need frequent blood tests (international normalized ratio or INR) to gauge your correct dose. The optimum INR for stroke prevention in atrial fibrillation is 2.0 to 3.0. However, the correct warfarin dose is affected by other drugs and by alcohol. Diet must also be fairly consistent, since the dose also depends on how much food rich in vitamin K you eat. Anyone taking warfarin must avoid contact sports, as an otherwise routine blow—such as a bodycheck or a crack on the head with a baseball—can cause fatal hemorrhage. It is also a good idea to switch to an electric shaver, because it will take longer to stem the flow of blood from a razor nick.

ASA also helps prevent some strokes in people with atrial fibrillation. Taking ASA is better than leaving atrial fibrillation untreated, but it is not nearly as effective as taking warfarin.

Electrical Cardioversion

If you have dangerously low blood pressure, severe angina or heart failure during atrial fibrillation, you may require emergency treatment in the form of an electrical shock to your chest to reset your heart rhythm to normal.

Electrical cardioversion may also be scheduled electively ("non-emergently"). When drug therapy has proven ineffective, an appointment is made for you to come to the hospital in the morning, undergo a cardioversion and return home later in the day.

After you sign a consent form, an anesthetist monitors your breathing and administers medications intravenously to cause a drug-induced coma. This comatose state lasts about five minutes and is followed by about an hour of mental haziness. While you are in the coma, two fluorescent orange, rubbery, rectangular pads are placed on your chest. One is typically to the right of the breastbone, and the other on the left side of the chest, just under the breast or below the armpit. These pads are used to "soften the blow" of the electrical shock.

Consent—to what?

If you undergo a cardioversion, you will be required to sign a consent form. Consent forms are used for many medical procedures to ensure that you understand and accept the risks and benefits of the procedure. While your consent ensures that you are making an informed decision, it will not protect a physician against negligence. If you enter the hospital for an electrical cardioversion and exit without your appendix, a signed consent will not get your physician off the hook—any more than it will get your appendix returned.

Rat poison

Warfarin can be used as rat poison; eaten in large enough doses, it causes rats (and other rodents) to bleed to death. Some alternative health care practitioners proclaim that warfarin is therefore part of a medical conspiracy to poison people. Science easily clears up this misconception, as the drug prevents more damage than it causes. Studies have shown that, if you were to treat 1,000 atrial fibrillation patients with warfarin for a year, and another 1,000 with a placebo, the group on warfarin would have a much better outcome. Of the people on the placebo, 41 would have a catastrophic, debilitating stroke. Of those on the warfarin, 15 would have a stroke and one or two would suffer a serious brain bleed. Which group would you rather be in? Thus, protests against the dangers of warfarin use should be ignored. They are often engineered by those interested in making a buck from an alternative and unproven product.

The shock is administered via a defibrillating machine, which is set for a certain amount of energy (anywhere from 25 to 360 joules). Two rectangular paddles are held by the cardiologist, and placed firmly on the chest over the orange rubber pads, a button is pushed to send a shock from one pad to the other, coursing through the heart. If the patient were conscious, the feeling would be comparable to being kicked in the chest by a horse. For the comatose patient, however, the shock goes completely unnoticed.

Since the electricity travels throughout the patient and even beyond, it's essential that nobody touches the patient (except via the shock-proof paddles) or the stretcher. More than one overly enthusiastic nurse, medical student or doctor has been inadvertently shocked through a dangling stethoscope touching the bed, or a hand resting on the stretcher.

The shock may be repeated two or three times in rapid succession if the first one doesn't reset the heart rhythm. In 5 to 10 percent of people, the atrial fibrillation is resistant to electrical cardioversion—most often when the condition has been present for more than a few months and/or the left atrium of the heart is enlarged.

There are other, more invasive cardioversion techniques that involve manipulating a catheter into the heart through a vein in the leg, and shocking the heart from the inside (with much less energy). This technique may prove necessary for someone who is very symptomatic and for whom no other treatment works.

Side Effects and Complications of Electrical Cardioversion
A common and innocuous side effect is a burning, itching sensation over the two rectangular areas on the chest wall, like a mild sunburn, that may last a few days. Imprints of the pads remain visible for a few days as well.

There is a very small chance that the heart will not reset after a shock, and that all electrical activity will cease—in other words, that the heart will stop (a condition called *asystole*). This is an emergency situation that requires urgent intervention. There is also a very small chance that the patient will suffer a stroke or die during the procedure. Patients who have had atrial fibrillation for less than forty-eight hours may undergo electrical cardioversion without prior medication. However, if you have had atrial fibrillation for more than forty-eight hours and you are not already taking warfarin, you should go on warfarin for four weeks prior to cardioversion, to minimize your stroke risk.

The risks associated with electrical cardioversion depend on the presence or absence of other problems. A ninety-five-year-old with diabetes, severe heart disease, lung and kidney ailments has a higher risk of complications than a fifty-year-old with no other medical problems.

Recent Advances
Recent large trials have raised questions about the usefulness of converting patients from atrial fibrillation into sinus rhythm, if they are medically stable and have minimal symptoms. Some

evidence suggests a higher risk of complications in people using anti-arrhythmic drugs, including sotalol, propafenone, flecainide and amiodarone. For years, doctors assumed that maintaining normal sinus rhythm reduced morbidity and mortality; reducing the heart rate during atrial fibrillation, instead of attempting pharmacological or electrical cardioversion, was viewed as an inferior option.

The recently published AFFIRM trial randomly divided people with atrial fibrillation into two groups. In the first group, heart rate during atrial fibrillation was controlled and no effort was made to convert it electrically. In the second group, combinations of drugs and electrical cardioversion were employed to maintain normal sinus rhythm.

At the conclusion of the study period, there had been more adverse events in the rhythm-control group than in the rate-control group, and a trend toward a higher mortality rate. This in part reflects the marginal success of anti-arrhythmic medications for this disorder, and their attendant risks. There was no difference in stroke incidence between the two groups.

This does not mean that people should simply accept atrial fibrillation without a fight. Up to 25 percent of patients continue to have significant symptoms with atrial fibrillation despite a controlled heart rate. Additionally, people having their first-ever episode of atrial fibrillation may benefit from attempts to use electrical cardioversion to restore sinus rhythm.

Margaret had been feeling unwell for the past week. She felt more tired than usual and had difficulty catching her breath. But at eighty-four, she figured she had a right to feel tired. Nevertheless, she had been healthy all her life, so she sought medical attention. After giving her doctor a history and having a physical, she was shocked to discover that she had atrial fibrillation.

"I suspect it started last week." her doctor surmised. "It explains why you're not feeling well. Your heart rate is a little too fast, but not excessive. Right now it's between 100 and 110. It should be about 70."

"Well, why don't I feel any palpitations or chest pain?" Margaret asked.

"It's not uncommon to have non-specific symptoms," her doctor told her. "Some patients sense every skipped beat, while others, like yourself, are unaware of the rhythm changes. I'd like to start you on a beta-blocker called metoprolol. It will slow down your heart rate, and it should give you more energy, although it causes fatigue in some people. I'll start you on a low dose today, and my secretary will arrange an appointment in two weeks to make sure your heart rate is controlled and you're feeling better. You'll also need to take warfarin. It's a blood thinner. It has no effect on the heart rhythm or rate, but it offers excellent protection against stroke resulting from atrial fibrillation. Your risk of a stroke is about 4 percent per year. With warfarin the risk is reduced to 1.5 percent per year."

After listening carefully to the doctor's explanation, Margaret decided to follow this advice. Within a week of starting the beta-blocker, her energy improved, although it never returned to normal.

Atrial Flutter

Atrial flutter is a less common arrhythmia. Like atrial fibrillation, it originates in the atrium. The number of electrical impulses is likewise excessive, but there are fewer impulses (usually 300 per minute) in atrial flutter than in atrial fibrillation and their production is more regular and organized. A person can have both atrial flutter and periods of atrial fibrillation. Atrial flutter is more likely to convert into either a regular rhythm or atrial fibrillation than persist as atrial flutter.

The treatment of atrial flutter is nearly identical to that of atrial fibrillation. Drugs work well to control the heart rate, but anti-arrhythmic therapy is even less effective than it is with atrial fibrillation. Electrical cardioversions are initially very successful, but not lasting.

A modern therapy for atrial flutter is radiofrequency catheter ablation (RFA), which is similar to an angiogram in preparation and technique. A catheter is placed in a leg vein (the femoral vein) to access the right side of the heart. The catheter locates the electrical abnormality and destroys it with precise high-energy radio waves, like a smart bomb. There is rarely collateral damage, but there are risks associated with the procedure. If the abnormality lies near the AV node, RFA may damage it, and one out of every 200 patients requires a permanent pacemaker. Other complications are even more rare.

Ventricular Tachycardia

Although heart attacks are the most common cause of cardiac damage, many other diseases may adversely affect the heart's function and cause electrical irritability. When a rapid heart rhythm begins in the ventricle it is called *ventricular tachycardia* (*VT*), a very bad rhythm to have. Although uncommon, VT occurs without warning, and it may first appear years after an initial cardiac incident such as a heart attack. In VT, an irritated and damaged ventricle suddenly initiates a heart rhythm itself, instead of awaiting instructions from its "master," the sinus node. A rapid and unstable rhythm may occur, with heart rates of up to 280 beats per minute. This instability is poorly tolerated, both because the heart rate is so rapid, and because patients who get VT are sicker and have weaker hearts. The heart barely has time to fill up with blood before another beat arrives. VT may cause low blood pressure, shortness of breath, chest pain, lightheadedness and even loss of consciousness (syncope).

Ventricular tachycardia may quickly degenerate into *ventricular fibrillation* (*VF*), a condition in which the heart quivers uncontrollably but does not beat effectively. Because VF produces no forward blood flow, if it is not reversed within minutes, brain damage and death will ensue. VT causes such instability that most people require an immediate electric shock, like the shock used for electrical conversion of atrial fibrillation.

Rare forms of ventricular tachycardia can occur in young people with otherwise healthy hearts. These people tend to be more stable, and to complain only of palpitations. In these cases, electrical cardioversion may not be immediately necessary, and VT may be treated in an emergency department with drugs.

When VT is brief (lasting less than thirty seconds) it's called *non-sustained* (*NSVT*). NSVT should always be investigated, even in the absence of symptoms, because it is often a marker for underlying cardiac disease. Once the acute episode has been treated, there are a number of options. Drugs such as beta-blockers and amiodarone can be used to stabilize electrical function, reducing the chances of further VT.

Some people on anti-arrhythmic therapy are eligible for a device called an *automatic implantable cardiac defibrillator* (*AICD*). This incredible piece of technology, which also serves as a pacemaker, is implanted through a vein into the heart, where it is sophisticated enough to recognize heart rhythms. When VT or VF is identified, the device delivers an internal shock to reset the heart. Whether it occurs in a hospital, on an airplane or in the middle of the Australian outback, an AICD can recognize and treat an arrhythmia. Not everyone with VT requires an AICD; the most suitable candidates include those with severe symptoms from the VT, such as fainting, and those with poor heart function.

Rhythm disturbances are a very common cardiac problem and compose a large slice of cardiology practice. Some are benign; others are terrifying. Although we have become adept at dealing with the emergencies, arrhythmias tend to recur, and medication options lag behind those available for other cardiac conditions.

Sudden Cardiac Death

Odd as it may sound, not everyone with *sudden cardiac death* (*SCD*) dies from it. SCD is defined as a sudden collapse within one hour of the onset of symptoms. Most people with SCD lose consciousness within one minute. Only 5 to 10 percent reach hospital in time and, of these, only half survive to be discharged. Of those who do survive an SCD episode, up to half are left with neurologic impairment. SCD accounts for 15 percent of all deaths in North America, becomes more common as we age and is two to three times more common in men than in women. Due to the high recurrence rate of sudden cardiac death, those who have survived an episode should be seriously considered for automatic implantable cardiac defibrillators.

Most people who suffer SCD already have an underlying cardiac condition, often coronary artery disease (CAD). Autopsy studies have demonstrated that 85 percent of people who die of out-of-hospital cardiac arrest show evidence of underlying coronary artery disease. In the absence of CAD, there may be a previously unrecognized structural ailment involving the muscle, valves or electrical system of the heart. Examples of these rare conditions include:

- hypertrophic cardiomyopathy (abnormally thick heart muscle)
- arrhythmogenic right ventricular dysplasia (abnormally thin right ventricle)
- long QT syndrome (rare electrical abnormality)
- Brugada syndrome (another rare electrical abnormality)
- various congenital heart defects

The younger the patient (age thirty-five is used as an arbitrary cutoff), the less likely it is that the origin of SCD is coronary artery disease.

A disturbance of heart rhythm—either abnormally fast or abnormally slow—is always present in SCD, and there is usually also an underlying heart problem, which the person may or may not be aware of. SCD may, rarely, occur in the absence of structural heart disease. If the person is fortunate enough to be rapidly resuscitated, the abnormal heart rhythm may be identified on a monitor during resuscitation efforts. Most of these rhythm abnormalities are tachycardias; abnormally slow rhythms are noted in only 10 percent of cases.

In SCD, ventricular tachycardia develops into ventricular fibrillation in thirty seconds to three minutes. Within four minutes of the collapse, 90 percent of patients have ventricular fibrillation, and the other 10 percent have a complete absence of any electrical activity. The most effective way to survive sudden death is to be lucky enough to have it in front of someone who knows CPR. The faster CPR is initiated, the greater the chance of survival.

Cardiopulmonary Resuscitation

When someone's heart stops beating, two processes that are essential to life come to a halt:

- breathing stops, so no fresh, oxygen-laden air enters the lungs;
- the blood that carries oxygen from the lungs to the brain and the rest of the body stops circulating.

Deprived of their oxygen supply, brain cells soon degrade and die.

Cardiopulmonary resuscitation (CPR) is a fairly simple maneuver to replace these two missing processes. It alternates mouth-to-mouth breathing, which puts oxygen-laden air into the lungs, with manual chest compressions, which pump the heart to send oxygen-bearing blood to the brain. CPR is a temporary first-aid measure—it rarely restarts the heart, and it's not efficient enough to sustain life for long. But in many cases it saves a life by keeping someone's brain alive until more advanced medical help arrives, usually with a defibrillator, to try to actually restart the person's heart.

Automatic External Defibrillators

An *automatic external defibrillator (AED)* is a portable, idiot-proof, battery-operated device that can be used by untrained bystanders. The AED is easily connected to an unconscious person. Once connected, the system itself recognizes rhythm abnormalities and displays instructions to the operator to push the "shock" button when indicated.

AEDs are very successful at rapidly restoring normal rhythm, but they carry a high price tag of about $3,000 U.S. Airports, malls and casinos are frequent sites of sudden cardiac death; accordingly, many of these facilities have elected to purchase AEDs. According to two published reports, approximately half the people treated with an AED by casino staff or airline attendants survived to be discharged from hospital. Government offices are other facilities where AEDs may be found (at taxpayers' expense).

Bill, a computer analyst, had received a wake-up call at the age of forty-eight. Back then, he'd been a smoker who paid little attention to his health. One morning, while taking out the garbage, he had suffered a heart attack. Fortunate to survive with only moderate heart damage, he had promised himself and his family that he would change his attitude and lifestyle.

Since that day, Bill had succeeded in modifying his risks with a combination of healthy eating, weight loss and exercise. He hadn't smoked a cigarette since his heart attack. At fifty, he was enjoying life more than ever.

Bill's exercise regimen included twice-weekly squash games. One morning, he and his partner, Warren, stretched and warmed up with a few minutes of practice shots and began to play. Minutes into the game, Bill lunged for the ball and suddenly collapsed on the court. Shocked at the sight of his squash partner unconscious and not breathing, Warren shouted for help.

Bill was lucky. A physician who was playing squash in a nearby court rushed over and began CPR without delay. Another player used his cellphone to call 911. While a small crowd of onlookers gathered, the doctor continued CPR. Within minutes, a paramedic team arrived. A monitor was attached to Bill and showed ventricular fibrillation. Within seconds, a 360-joule shock of electricity shot through paddles placed on Bill's chest, making his body lurch upwards. The squash court was quiet. After a few seconds, the monitor showed a normal rhythm. Bill's pulse and blood pressure had been restored; he was still unconscious but he was breathing on his own. A dose of lidocaine (an anti-arrhythmic drug) was injected, and Bill was put on oxygen and transported to the nearest emergency room. He had suffered sudden cardiac death, and he had survived.

7. Congestive Heart Failure

Congestive heart failure (CHF) is the most common reason for hospitalization in North America of people over sixty-five years of age. It is the only major cardiac disease that is becoming more common. For some people, the prognosis is worse than it is for most cancers.

Heart function is graded on a four-point scale based on the appearance of the muscle on ultrasound. Normal heart function is grade 1/4 (one out of four, not one quarter). Severe weakness is grade 4/4. Mild or moderate weakness is between 2/4 and 3/4. Weakness of the heart muscle, regardless of the cause, is called *cardiomyopathy*. When someone begins to experience symptoms of a weak heart, the diagnosis is *congestive heart failure* (CHF).

The heart is a pump. Damage to the pump makes it harder to propel the blood forward. Like water in a plugged drainpipe, the blood will then back up toward where it came from: the lungs and the rest of the body. But because the blood has nowhere to go, pressure builds, causing the *plasma* (the liquid component of the blood, not the actual blood cells) to leak through the blood vessel walls into the lungs. Leakage may also occur into other tissue. Because of gravity, swelling of the feet and legs is common, as the fluid settles into parts closest to the ground. Fluid overload is typical of CHF, although it can also occur in other conditions.

NYHA classification of congestive heart failure

Symptoms of heart failure are classified according to a simple four-point system, the New York Heart Association (NYHA) system.

Class I—no limitation of activities

Class II—slight limitation of activities, mild shortness of breath with ordinary activities

Class III—marked limitation of activities, shortness of breath with minimal exertion

Class IV—severe symptoms, shortness of breath at rest or with any activity

Leakage into the lungs is called *pulmonary edema.* This is an anxiety-provoking ailment; it has been described as a sensation of running quickly, unable to slow your pace to catch your breath. Breathing difficulties predominate and fatigue is common. In the early stages shortness of breath begins with minimal exertion, and ultimately occurs at rest. This shortness of breath is reduced in an upright position and made worse by lying flat, a symptom called *orthopnea.* (*Orthos* is Greek for "upright"; *pnoe* is Greek for "air.") The reason for this orthopnea is simple. When you are upright, the top portions of your lungs remain air-filled and are unaffected by the leaking fluid. When you are lying flat, however, gravity distributes the fluid throughout your lungs, resulting in fewer "dry" areas to aerate. Another frightening symptom is *paroxysmal nocturnal dyspnea* (PND). This ominous term means suddenly awakening from sleep with marked breathlessness. (Waking up to urinate in the middle of the night [nocturia] isn't a symptom of heart failure.)

Causes of Congestive Heart Failure

What causes CHF? What weakens the heart? The most common cause is large heart attacks. The second most common cause is chronic hypertension (high blood pressure). The heart has a limited capacity to generate excessively high blood pressures before it gives up. It's like the World's Strongest Man Contest: the winner is the one who can hold up the front end of a car longest, but even the strongest man eventually drops it. Some CHF is described as *idiopathic*, a fancy way of saying "we have absolutely no idea what caused this." (This term is applied to many diseases, to lend a knowledgeable air to current medical ignorance.)

Idiopathic heart failure is probably viral in origin, but this diagnosis is difficult to prove. We are all exposed to hundreds of viruses in our lives. Rarely, a common cold or stomach virus attacks and weakens the heart. When someone with no other cause of heart failure has a weak heart, it's hard to diagnose an infection that may be long past. As a result, the bin of "idiopathic and presumably viral" diagnoses becomes filled with these cases. Although most causes of idiopathic heart failure are probably viral, many are simply unknown.

It is important for the physician to obtain a detailed alcohol history of anyone with unexplained heart failure. Alcoholics are more likely to develop CHF, as alcohol is toxic to muscle tissue. Because it has been shown that alcoholics are rarely honest about their drinking history, medical school cynically teaches students to multiply a patient's reported alcohol intake by three, to arrive at a truer amount. Many people claim to drink alcohol "socially," but the definition of social drinking is subjective; for some it's a few beers per week, and for others it's a few beers per hour.

Other Causes of Cardiomyopathy

Aside from the reasons mentioned above—heart attacks, high blood pressure, viruses, excessive alcohol consumption—there are other causes of heart weakness:

- valve disease
- legal drugs (some chemotherapy and, rarely, other medications)
- illegal drugs (cocaine)
- nutritional deficiency (of thiamine, selenium, carnitine)
- endocrine conditions (thyroid, diabetes and others)
- infections (viruses such as HIV, bacterial diseases and more)
- collagen vascular diseases (lupus, scleroderma, dermatomyositis)
- sarcoidosis (a rare inflammatory condition that can cause scar tissue in almost any organ of the body)
- amyloidosis (a rare condition of amyloid deposits)
- post-pregnancy cardiomyopathy
- heredity

Education

As with many conditions, people with CHF live longer when they understand their disease. Self-management of heart failure is simple, but it calls for a multidisciplinary approach, involving physicians, nurses, dietitians and others. To turn congestive heart failure (CHF) into congestive heart success (CHS), patients are regularly reviewed in the clinic, and have access to the nurse or doctor at almost any time. If you are suffering symptoms, you can get medical attention the same day if necessary. This accessible approach not only eases the anxiety of the patient and family and promotes confidence, but has also been shown to improve survival rates and reduce hospitalization. A CHF clinic should be part of every major hospital.

Cold winter weather is associated with an increased risk of hospitalization for heart failure. (This is a very good excuse to head south with the first sign of frost!) The reason for the increase is likely the greater risk of lung infections during cold weather, and our tendency to exercise less when snow and ice cover the ground. When someone's cardiac function is tenuous, it can take very little stress to exacerbate heart failure symptoms.

Salt (Na+) and Water (H₂O) Intake

In CHF, the weakened heart muscle has trouble pumping blood forward. This problem leads to a unique downward spiral. The kidneys, like all organs in the body, rely on the heart for blood supply. If the heart can't fulfill this simple task, the kidneys perceive that there is an inadequate blood *volume*. The kidneys have no idea that they are "seeing" less blood because the heart isn't working well. As far as they are concerned, the lack of blood flow might be from blood loss through bleeding, or from dehydration. Regardless of why there is less flow (bad heart or massive bleeding), the kidneys respond by releasing hormones to inhibit urine formation, forcing the body to retain water and salt. Already overworked and faced with too much blood to pump, the weak heart suddenly faces even more work. The system becomes overwhelmed, and liquid seeps into the lungs and lower limbs (again, because of gravity). If this situation continues long enough, the whole body becomes saturated with fluid—a condition called *anasarca*. Fluid overload, although a hallmark of CHF, can occur in various other medical conditions.

How do we combat this cycle? There are drug approaches and non-drug approaches. All forms of liquid intake, whether a can of pop or a bowl of soup, must be reduced, as any liquids will be absorbed from the gut into the bloodstream and will further overload the system. However, it's important not to become obsessive about liquid. Monitoring is necessary, but occasional lapses are understandable; it makes no sense to spend the day thirsty and uncomfortable. Your particular liquid "prescription" from your cardiologist will depend on your symptoms and the severity of your heart failure. A typical recommendation is no more than 1.5 quarts (liters) per twenty-four hours. For some people, this may be too much. Each person must find a balance between the dryness of the desert and the spray of the ocean.

Excess sodium is another no-no for people with CHF. Although sodium is an important mineral, essential for normal functioning, too much is harmful for those with weak hearts. Salt, and the water that accompanies it, is absorbed by the intestine. High salt intake thus aggravates heart failure and may cause short-term and long-term problems. The only way to limit salt intake is to know where it is. Throwing away the salt shaker won't be enough, as most of the salt we eat is present in foods before they reach the dinner table. Reading packages helps determine the salt content of most foods. Any listing containing the word sodium should be scrutinized. Swimming in salty water is fine, as long as your mouth remains closed.

Medications for CHF
Drugs form the cornerstone of CHF management. Combinations of medications allow people with CHF to live longer, with fewer hospitalizations and fewer symptoms. Important drugs include beta-blockers, ACE inhibitors, various diuretics ("water pills") and nitroglycerin.

CHF and Monitoring Weight
People with CHF must weigh themselves every day. The only reliable method is to weigh yourself first thing in the morning, naked (light underwear is allowed), after you have emptied your bladder but before you eat or drink. Minor daily increases in weight are usually due to fluid retention. If your weight slowly creeps up over the week, due to fluid retention, the change is often accompanied by initially mild symptoms, such

as lack of energy, leg swelling and subtle shortness of breath. Instead of waiting until your symptoms become desperate, increase the amount of diuretic you are taking and further reduce your salt and fluid intake. This early self-management may help you avoid the need for hospitalization or even a visit to the doctor. Self-management is emphasized in specialized CHF clinics, which provide telephone assessments to guide home treatment.

After two months of fatigue and breathlessness, Andrew knew something was amiss. His illness had crept up on him like a tickle in the throat. He was developing progressive shortness of breath with less and less activity. At first it had taken a flight of stairs to trouble him. Then just taking out the garbage and rushing out the door in the morning had left him gasping. He had attributed his symptoms to work and family stress, but he had a desk job at the post office, and at fifty-nine years of age he was near retirement. His marriage was happy and his three children had long since moved out on their own.

Andrew kept trying to deny the obvious, but one Friday evening he and his wife, Marie, decided to order in Chinese food. After stuffing himself with salty offerings, he retired to the den to watch TV with Marie. Within thirty minutes his breathing worsened, and he felt as if he were in the midst of a long, arduous jog. He couldn't catch his breath, and his coughing was incessant. Gripped by fear, he motioned to the phone. "Call 911," he ordered his frightened wife.

Andrew had never before experienced his symptoms at rest. Although he tried to remain calm, a sense of doom enveloped him. The ambulance arrived within seven minutes, by which time he was in extreme respiratory distress and unable to talk. Because breathlessness puts tremendous strain on the muscles of breathing, Andrew's muscles were having difficulty maintaining the rapid respiratory rate he needed to ensure adequate oxygenation of his blood. The paramedics recognized that without immediate action their patient would be dead.

A tube was inserted through Andrew's nose, across his trachea and into his lungs. Clear liquid bubbled up from his lungs and through the tube. The tube was connected to a tank of 100 percent oxygen, and the medic rhythmically pumped air into Andrew's lungs via a balloon-like "ambu" bag. This let the paramedics take over the work of Andrew's breathing.

With an intravenous line in place, the medics injected 80 milligrams of furosemide, a diuretic, into Andrew's veins to promote fluid removal via his kidneys. Most of this fluid would come from his congested lungs. At the same time, 2 milligrams of morphine was administered to calm him, and a transdermal patch of nitroglycerin was placed on his arm to help relieve his lung congestion by dilating his blood vessels, so that blood could more easily flow away from his lungs.

The entire treatment took seventeen minutes. By the time the group arrived at the hospital five minutes later, Andrew's condition had significantly improved. He was admitted to the intensive care unit with a diagnosis of acute congestive heart failure, and placed on a ventilator (breathing machine). The following day, the endotracheal tube was removed and he was taken off the ventilator.

Surrounded by his family, Andrew sat up in bed and polished off a small tub of Jell-O. He still had no idea what had gone wrong. A middle-aged doctor came in and explained what had transpired.

"Your heart had become extremely weak, and after your large meal it was unable to continue pumping all your blood through your body. So some of the blood's plasma, the liquid component, leaked into your lungs."

Marie was confused. "Why is his heart weak?" she asked.

"I can't be sure yet," the doctor said. "It's most likely because of either a previously unrecognized heart attack, or a virus. Since you don't take drugs or drink alcohol and you don't suffer from high blood pressure, these causes don't seem to apply to you. I'm going to have the heart failure clinic nurse visit you prior to discharge to go over some of the dos and don'ts, and I'll see you next week in the clinic."

Andrew's doctor recommended that, because a weakened heart muscle is occasionally hereditary, Andrew's children should undergo precautionary echocardiograms to evaluate their heart function. In addition, he increased Andrew's medications, set him up for further testing, and established his care in the congestive heart failure clinic, where Andrew learned about dietary restrictions and the importance of taking medication conscientiously.

Andrew's heart never recovered its strength; he remained more fatigued than in the past. But he adhered to his diet and tolerated his medications, and he and Marie continued to lead an active life during their retirement.

8. Valve Disease and Valve Surgery

The valves in the heart ensure that blood flows through the heart in only one direction. Like a door that shuts behind you after you pass through it, the valves keep the blood moving forward.

The two valves on the left side of the heart (the mitral and aortic valves) are more important than the two on the right (the tricuspid and pulmonary), so diseases of the mitral and aortic valves are more serious. The mitral valve connects the left atrium to the left ventricle. The valve derives its name from its resemblance to a mitre, a folding hat used by Catholic popes, bishops and cardinals. The aortic valve is the final crossing point for blood as it exits the left ventricle and is propelled into the aorta to be circulated through the body. On the other side of the heart, the tricuspid valve lies between the right atrium and right ventricle, while the pulmonic valve separates the right ventricle from the pulmonary artery, which leads to the lungs.

The mitral and tricuspid valves look alike, and resemble parachutes with central holes opening and closing. The aortic and pulmonic valves also look alike; each has three

119

cusps (leaflets) opening and closing. Viewed from above, the aortic and pulmonic valves look somewhat like the insignia on a Mercedes-Benz, which many cardiac surgeons probably drive.

Valves of the heart

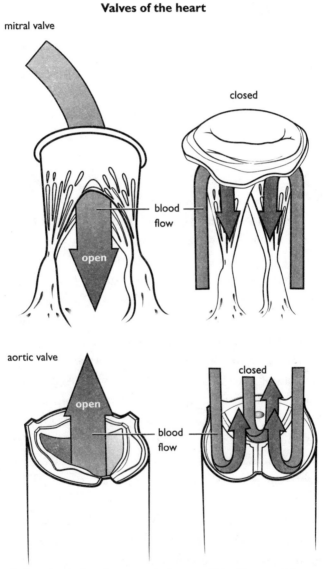

When the heart beats, the valves are pushed open and blood is pumped forward. The valves open in only one direction, ensuring that blood does not flow back again.

A normal heart beats about 100,000 times a day and the valves open and close each time, so they have to be remarkably durable. Like a spider web with the tensile strength of the strongest steel, valves are constructed of three thin layers of connective-tissue proteins called *elastin* and *collagen*. Even so, over the two or three billion openings and closings of an average lifespan, it is no wonder that some valves fail. In fact, it's amazing that so many don't.

There are only two types of valve complications; leaky (regurgitant) valves and narrow (stenotic) valves. Any one or more of the four valves can be too leaky or too narrow or, often, both leaky and narrow. Pulmonary valve disease and tricuspid stenosis are uncommon conditions.

A *regurgitant* valve will not close properly; this is what causes the leakiness. Instead of moving forward, some of the blood moves backward. The amount of backward blood flow determines whether the leakiness is mild, moderate or severe. Mild regurgitation is common and in most cases it does not get worse, but the problem should be periodically reviewed. Moderate or severe regurgitation is a greater concern, depending on which valve is affected. If there is no immediate indication for surgery, severe valve disease should be closely monitored many times a year.

A *stenotic* valve is like a partially closed door; it does not allow enough blood to move forward. Because insufficient blood flows to the body, people with significant valvular stenosis easily become fatigued and breathless. There are different degrees of narrowing, with the most severe narrowing causing the most trouble.

An echocardiogram can not only diagnose valvular abnormalities but can also evaluate their severity. All valve disease, whether regurgitation or stenosis, is categorized as trace, mild, moderate or severe, based on echocardiography, the single most important test in the recognition and evaluation of valve disease.

Mitral Valve

Mitral Regurgitation

A regurgitant mitral valve can be *secondary to* many different diseases, meaning that the valve itself is not the problem. If the heart is enlarged (dilated), the valve leaflets may not fit together well. Imagine an expanding door frame—the door itself is still normal, but the house around it is too big. The problem is progressive: the larger the heart becomes, the more the mitral valve leaks; the more the mitral valve leaks, the larger the heart will become. Unfortunately, someone with a weak, dilated heart and severe mitral regurgitation may not be able to withstand surgery. These patients have few tenable operative options.

Diseases that affect the mitral valve itself may cause *primary* mitral regurgitation. There are many types of this condition. One is *mitral valve prolapse (MVP)*, in which the valve is thick and there is excessive "floppy" valve tissue. As a result, each time the mitral valve closes, a portion of it moves into the left atrium, creating an opening for blood to move backward. Although MVP is common, it rarely progresses to become clin-

Rheumatic fever and heart disease

Rheumatic fever is caused by the effects of a bacterial throat infection that often occurs in childhood. Rheumatic heart disease has dramatically declined in North America, due to improved medical care and the use of antibiotics, but it remains common in Third World countries. When the body fights the throat infection, it inadvertently damages the heart valves. This damage progresses over a period of decades, after the infection is long gone. Eventually, over many years, manifestations of the damage include leaky and/or narrowed heart valves, along with mitral regurgitation.

ically important. It is only important when it is associated with more than mild regurgitation.

As well, the mitral valve can be affected by bacterial infections, which are a rare cause of regurgitation. Heart valve infection (*endocarditis*) more often occurs in a valve that is already abnormal. Valve problems can also result from rheumatic fever.

Mitral regurgitation can occur after certain types of heart attacks. When the inferior (lower) and/or posterior (back) walls of the heart have been damaged, the supporting structure of the mitral valve may be injured, resulting in mitral regurgitation. Shortness of breath and fatigue are more likely to occur in someone whose heart attack has resulted in mitral regurgitation.

Over time, mitral regurgitation can worsen, weakening the heart. It can also cause a build-up of fluid in the lungs (pulmonary edema). Although there are medications for treating mitral regurgitation, they merely delay the inevitable surgery and do not cure the problem. While they may act to minimally reduce the slope of decline, regurgitation persists. The only cure is surgery, to either replace or, preferably, repair the leaky mitral valve.

Mitral Stenosis

In North America, mitral stenosis is less common than mitral regurgitation, although both conditions can occur in the same person. Almost all cases of mitral stenosis are due to rheumatic fever causing rheumatic heart disease, and most cases in North America are diagnosed in people who immigrated from other countries.

In this condition, blood flowing from the left atrium to the left ventricle has to pass through a narrowed mitral valve. In the early stages of the disease, symptoms only occur during physical exertion, when more blood is required. Unfortunately, mitral stenosis is a progressive disease, and as it becomes more severe it causes difficulty breathing during less and less exertion. The more severe the stenosis, the worse the symptoms. As with congestive heart failure, the New York Heart Association classification is used to describe the severity of symptoms.

Pulmonary hypertension—increased blood pressure within the lungs—is a serious potential consequence of mitral stenosis. Normal blood pressure in the pulmonary artery is 35 mm/Hg. (This can be measured during an echocardiogram, or as part of a heart catheterization.) When pulmonary hypertension complicates mitral stenosis, surgery is often necessary, even if the symptoms are minimal.

It's important that mitral stenosis be identified long before pulmonary hypertension develops. The stenosis is usually treated by mitral valve replacement when the person begins to notice symptoms. There are less invasive techniques for treating mitral stenosis. In *valvuloplasty*, which is available in specialized cardiac centers, a balloon is passed across the valve and inflated, widening the valve opening and improving the blood flow. However, valvuloplasty is appropriate in only a few selected cases, and should be undertaken only by specialized cardiologists, of whom there are few.

Medications cannot cure mitral stenosis. Diuretics and beta-blockers may reduce the symptoms, but without valve surgery the inexorable decline will continue. The stenosis distorts the structure of the left atrium, which may be massively dilated in people with severe mitral stenosis. This enlargement promotes atrial arrhythmias—most important, atrial fibrillation. The combination of mitral stenosis and atrial fibrillation raises the risk of stroke dramatically. Warfarin effectively lowers the risk of stroke. In fact, some authorities consider severe mitral stenosis with left atrial enlargement to be in itself an indication for warfarin use, even in the absence of atrial fibrillation.

Tricuspid Valve

Tricuspid Regurgitation

Tricuspid regurgitation (TR) is a common valve abnormality. Unlike mitral or aortic valve disease, tricuspid valve problems do not frequently require major intervention—partly because blood pressures are lower on the right side of the heart, where the tricuspid valve is located, and lower pressures translate into a reduced capacity to do damage. Tricuspid regurgitation may be secondary to high blood pressures in the lungs (pulmonary hypertension), which occur in people with various forms of lung disease, the most common of which are smoking-related.

The tricuspid is the valve closest to the front of the chest, so chest trauma from any cause, including motor vehicle accidents, can seriously damage the valve and cause sudden severe TR. When TR develops suddenly, instead of progressing over decades, it is more likely to require surgery.

Mild or moderate TR causes no symptoms. Moderate TR should be monitored yearly, but mild TR does not require regular follow-up. Symptoms of severe TR include fatigue, breathlessness during activities and leg swelling (edema). Most people with TR are able to tolerate the condition, and don't require surgical correction. However, some develop critical weakness of the right ventricle after years of severe tricuspid regurgitation, and may require a heart transplant.

Aortic Valve

Aortic Stenosis

Aortic stenosis (AS), one of the most common valve diseases, is a progressive narrowing of the aortic valve that restricts blood flow more and more. Most people with AS are in their late sixties and seventies. A common cause of AS is age-related valvular degeneration (known as Monckberg's sclerosis); all body parts eventually break down, and the aortic valve is no exception.

The most common symptoms of AS are fatigue, breathlessness with minimal activity, chest pain, lightheadedness and loss of consciousness. Over months to years the shortness of breath becomes worse, appearing with less and less activity. Another common complaint of people with aortic stenosis is angina. As less blood moves across the valve, the heart must work harder to meet the needs of the body. Ultimately too much work is required, and chest pain results. Less often, people develop lightheadedness with exertion; rarely, they collapse and lose consciousness. The most serious complication of aortic stenosis is congestive heart failure.

Some people are born with two (bicuspid) instead of three (tricuspid) aortic valve leaflets, and they are more likely to suffer from AS. Because of their missing leaflet, blood flows across the valve and creates turbulence around the thin leaflets, which leads to further damage and narrowing of the valve. Aortic stenosis from a bicuspid valve occurs decades earlier than degenerative aortic stenosis.

Aortic stenosis may be diagnosed after symptoms develop, but it is more often recognized during a routine physical examination. It causes a loud "murmur." Many people have benign, physiologic murmurs. Pregnant women, for example, almost always have murmurs, even although their heart valves are almost always perfectly normal. The nature of the murmur, including its pitch, loudness and location, indicates whether it represents a valve disorder. A good doctor will be able to tell whether a murmur requires further investigation with a cardiac ultrasound test (echocardiogram).

Because there is no drug therapy for aortic stenosis, the only treatment option is surgical valve replacement; the natural valve is replaced by either a mechanical or a bioprosthetic valve (from a human or animal). Only rarely can the valve be repaired rather than replaced.

Not all cardiac surgeons have expertise in every cardiovascular surgical procedure. If valve surgery is recommended by your cardiologist, it is wise to get a referral to a surgeon who specializes in your particular valvular problem.

Aortic Regurgitation

The aortic valve may also become leaky. Aortic regurgitation (AR) may exist independently, or it may develop in association with aortic stenosis. Like mitral regurgitation, aortic regurgitation overloads the heart muscle with blood, making it work harder and harder. With every contraction of the heart muscle, blood is propelled forward through the aorta. If the valve is leaky, a portion of forward flow returns to the left ventricle, joining the blood destined for the next heartbeat. This is very inefficient, as the heart must make up for the blood leaking backwards by propelling even more blood forwards. Over time, this extra volume of blood strains the left ventricle of the heart, causing it to enlarge and ultimately weaken.

Severe aortic regurgitation may be acute (beginning suddenly), but more often it develops over years. In acute AR, the heart has no time to adjust to the sudden backflow of large volumes of blood. Instead of flowing back into a bigger reser-

Echocardiography

Echocardiography is very useful and very remunerative, two reasons why its use has exploded in the last decade. Because it's such a profitable test, some unscrupulous laboratories (and doctors) perform it with inadequate expertise and a lack of quality control. Unfortunately, it can be difficult to gauge just how bad a valve condition is, especially for a non-expert. It is very important to ensure that your echocardiogram is performed in a reputable laboratory by a cardiologist.

voir, enlarged by years of progressive regurgitation, the blood moves into a normal left ventricle that doesn't have room for the added volume. This results in congestive heart failure, and is a life-threatening emergency. People with acute severe AR require emergency valve replacement, a procedure that carries a relatively high complication rate when performed emergently. Causes of acute aortic regurgitation include valvular infection (endocarditis), tearing (dissection) of the aorta and trauma.

More commonly, severe aortic regurgitation is chronic, advancing over many years. The murmur of AR should be detected by your physician during a physical examination, leading to an echocardiogram. The "echo" will help determine the severity of the AR.

Symptoms of chronic severe AR, like those of many valve diseases, are predominantly respiratory. Breathlessness during exertion is usually an early and constant symptom of chronic severe AR, but unfortunately it is not specific to valvular or, for that matter, cardiac disease. The very existence of progressive shortness of breath accompanying severe aortic regurgitation is an indication for surgical valve replacement. Less often, someone may have severe AR and have no symptoms. In these cases, the echo is used to determine the appropriate time for surgical intervention. If the left ventricle begins to show dilation or weakness on echocardiography, even without shortness of breath, valve replacement is indicated. For this reason, anyone with aortic regurgitation should be closely monitored from one to four times per year, depending on the circumstances.

Aortic and mitral regurgitation are both causes of heart failure and of fluid build-up in the lungs. Dozens of different diseases can contribute to the development of chronic severe AR, including high blood pressure. Medication is of marginal benefit; again, the best treatment option is surgery.

Valve Surgery

Valve surgery can be a lengthy procedure, which increases the risk of complications. Although heart valves can be either replaced or repaired, repairing is always preferable, because replaced valves expose the patient to a new set of potential problems with far greater frequency, including valvular failure and infections. Therefore, as much normal valve anatomy as possible should be left in place. Whereas mitral valves can often be repaired, however, aortic valve abnormalities are less amenable to repair and are usually replaced. Some people need both the aortic and the mitral valve replaced, which significantly increases the mortality rate, especially if coronary bypass is also needed.

Sometimes the decision to repair or replace cannot be made until the surgeon sees the valvular structure during the surgery. Even if the plan is to repair the valve, the task may be too difficult, and an unexpected replacement may be necessary.

It is routine for the surgeon to order a coronary angiogram prior to valve surgery, for anyone at risk of coronary artery disease (any man over forty and every woman over fifty). This is because CAD may be present without symptoms. Knowing whether bypass surgery will be needed at the same time as the valve surgery reduces the risk of a heart attack during the surgery, and the chance that a bypass will be required shortly after the valve surgery. "Redo surgery" on the heart is associated with twice the complication rate of the original surgery (valve replacement or bypass).

A valve may be replaced with either a tissue prosthesis—a human or animal valve—or a mechanical one. However, there are not enough human valves (*homografts*) available for widespread use. Accordingly, a cow or pig tissue prosthesis (*heterograft*) may be used. Just as an observant Hindu would not accept a cow prosthesis, an Orthodox Jew would not want a prosthesis made from pig tissue.

Mechanical valves come in many varieties. They may be named for the hospital that created them (such as St. Jude's valves) or, more commonly, the engineer and surgeon who teamed up in their design (Bjork-Shiley, Carpentier-Edwards, etc.). Composed of durable materials, St. Jude's valves are made of graphite coated in pyrolytic carbon; they are very expensive, costing thousands of dollars each.

Valves go through a lengthy quality control process, including animal experiments, to ensure safety before they are approved for use in humans. Despite this rigorous testing, in the mid-1980s too many patients with a particular type of Bjork-Shiley valve were dying suddenly. The valve was composed of two parts welded together, and it was discovered that one part was coming off, like a wing coming off an airplane, with similar catastrophic consequences. The manufacturing process was quickly modified and the valve was produced as a single unit.

Valves from animals and humans (bioprosthetics) are less durable than mechanical valves and more likely to deteriorate over time. However, the body considers a mechanical valve to be foreign material, and as a result, blood clots form on the valve, obstructing the valve orifice, a rapidly fatal condition. It's vital for people with mechanical valves to pay close attention to their warfarin dose, to thin the blood and prevent these clots. Bioprosthetic valves do not require lifelong warfarin, as they infrequently develop blood clots on their surface.

When a patient takes warfarin, a blood test known as the INR reflects how thin the blood is. The higher the INR, the less able the body is to form clots. In people with mechanical valves the INR should be 2.5 to 3.5, to prevent clots from forming on the valve surface.

Cardiac valves can be damaged in many ways. Most people with valve disease have only a small amount of leakiness or narrowing, and the damage does not usually progress. When treatment is required, however, medication does little, while surgery is curative. It's up to the cardiologist to follow cases of valve disease attentively, and identify the appropriate time for surgery, if necessary.

Mitchell was a vigorous and active man of seventy-six. However, his symptoms of breathlessness were getting worse. He was still jogging up to 2 miles (3 km) per day, but he was clocking himself at slower times, and he noticed shortness of breath and light-headedness if he pushed himself.

Mitchell's family doctor listened intently to his history, and noted that his patient had last been reviewed two years ago, at which time a heart murmur had been detected: when a stethoscope was pressed against Mitchell's chest, the doctor had heard the blood moving across the heart valves. At the time, he believed the murmur to be benign, and did not feel an echocardiogram was called for.

This time, when the doctor listened to Mitchell's chest, he knew this was not a benign murmur. It was very loud, very long and very harsh, all indications of aortic stenosis.

"It sounds as if one of your valves is narrowed. The symptoms you're complaining of would fit with a narrowed valve, but they aren't too specific, so I'd like to arrange a couple of tests."

An echocardiogram confirmed the doctor's suspicion. Mitchell had severe aortic stenosis with a valve area of 0.7 cm^2 (normal is 3 to 4 cm^2). The opening of the aortic valve was so tight that not enough blood was exiting the heart to meet the body's needs. The reduction in blood flow led to Mitchell's symptoms of increasing shortness of breath on exertion, and lightheadedness.

There are many heart drugs that should be used cautiously, if at all, in patients with significant aortic stenosis. They may worsen symptoms and can be dangerous. These include the angiotensin converting enzyme inhibitor (ACEIs), angiotensin receptor blockers (ARBs) and some calcium-channel blockers (nifedipine and amlodipine). The only available treatment for severe aortic stenosis is replacement of the aortic valve. Because of his age, Mitchell had a coronary angiogram before the operation to check that his blood vessels did not require a bypass at the same time as the valve replacement. Within a month of diagnosis of his valve problem, he underwent successful aortic valve replacement with a bioprosthetic valve. Six weeks after surgery, he was exercising at the gym, running three miles a day.

9. Rehabilitation, Diet and Sex

The concept of cardiac rehabilitation, which was initiated almost forty years ago, is simple. Collect a large group of patients with some form of coronary artery disease, teach them about their condition, start them on a supervised exercise program and hope they continue to follow a healthy lifestyle when the program is finished.

The main thrust of modern rehabilitation programs is education. There are weekly lectures during a six-month to twelve-month program, during which heart disease is reviewed, risk factors are identified and an approach to heart-healthy living is taught.

Cardiac rehab programs are very effective, and have been shown to reduce death rates and hospitalizations from recurrent heart disease. People feel better and are much more functional, with a greater percentage rejoining the workforce compared to similar patients who did not attend rehab. Cardiac rehab programs also save the government money, by reducing health care expenditures.

Unfortunately, only about one in five eligible patients attends cardiac rehab after suffering a heart attack, or having angioplasty or bypass surgery. Part of the explanation is that some patients are simply unwilling to participate. A larger part of the problem is the failure of health care providers to consider rehab an important component of treatment. Rehabilitation is not high-tech and exciting enough for many doctors, despite the incredible satisfaction that patients derive from the process. Many of us just plain forget to recommend it to our patients.

Diet

Innumerable diet books have been penned. Like religion, they all claim they will guide us down the true path. Too many diets are fad-based, however, focusing on cabbage for a month or celery for a year. The fundamental principle of an effective diet is fewer calories and less "bad" fat. There are more than twice as many calories in fat (9 calories per gram) as in the same weight of protein or carbohydrates (4 calories per gram).

A major impediment to following dietary recommendations is understanding the advice. Restricting your intake to 400 mg of this and 1,200 calories of that is difficult. Advice and direction must be meaningful to you to be useful.

A "heart-healthy" diet will promote weight loss, reduce your blood cholesterol and reduce your heart attack risk. It includes limited fat, but fat should still be part of the diet, since some fat is essential for normal body function. Very low-fat diets may lower cholesterol, but they require serious motivation and they are not very palatable. Evidence suggests that such diets may actually raise triglycerides and do not contain

---

Fundamental principles of a heart-healthy diet

1. Eat fewer calories.
2. Know the fat content of everything that goes into your mouth.
3. Know how much fat you should be eating.
4. Know which fats are good for your heart and which are not.

enough vitamins. Very low-fat diets are *not* the first step in the dietary management of heart disease and high cholesterol.

Here are some specific dietary "commandments" for those with heart disease:

1. Don't eat butter (which is almost all bad fat).
2. Don't eat foods cooked with butter.
3. Don't even look at butter.
4. Don't eat liver or animal skin (very high in bad fat). Cooking chicken with the skin on and removing it after preparation is useless; the fat melts into the meat.
5. Don't eat regular ice cream. It is high in fat; sorbet is not.
6. Eat fish (high in good fat) without cream sauces.
7. Don't eat cream sauces.
8. Don't cook with oils (even "healthy oils"); cooking turns the oil into bad fat.
9. Read labels of packaged meats to see how much fat is present. Some meats are truly lean; others are not.
10. Eat fruits and vegetables.
11. Embrace fiber; it lowers cholesterol.
12. Avoid processed and packaged foods; most contain hydrogenated vegetable oil, partially hydrogenated vegetable oil and transfatty acids. These are potent artery cloggers and very bad fat.
13. Don't frequent fast food outlets.
14. Don't eat cheese that is very high in saturated fat.
15. Eat beans. They are good for your heart.

Sex

Although some people want more of it and some want less, those who initiate the discussion in the doctor's office usually want the former. Heart patients often question their cardiologists about the stress of sexual activity on the heart. Understandably, they fear the possibility of having a heart attack

Risk of sex-related heart attack

If you have any of the following conditions, your risk of sex-related heart attack is:

Low:
- controlled hypertension
- mild and stable angina
- uncomplicated heart attack more than six weeks previously
- after successful bypass or angioplasty

Intermediate:
- moderate although stable angina
- heart attack two to six weeks previously
- moderately symptomatic heart failure

High:
- severe angina
- uncontrolled hypertension
- severe heart failure
- heart attack within past two weeks
- other significant heart disease

during sex. Fortunately, the risk is extremely low. As a rule of thumb, if you can perform a treadmill test without angina or serious difficulties, you can safely partake in other less strenuous activities.

In a study of 1,600 heart attack survivors, 27 had engaged in sexual intercourse within two hours before the event. Sex had contributed to the heart attack in less than 1 percent of cases. Statistically, if a person is at a "clinically low risk" of a heart attack—meaning that he or she can complete a treadmill test, for example—the risk of a heart attack is about 1 percent per year. If that same person has sex (assuming it is not too extreme) once a week, the risk goes up to 1.01 percent. To most people, this seems like a reasonable trade-off. If the person has regular angina and is considered to have a higher cardiac risk, the chance of a heart attack rises to 1.2 percent per year.

In most cases, sexual intercourse is just not that extreme an exertion. When people were monitored during sex (a somewhat unusual study design), those who did not show low blood flow to the heart during a treadmill test did not show low blood flow during sex either.

Viagra and Nitroglycerin

Sildenafil (sold under the brand name Viagra) has become immensely popular among men as a treatment for erectile dysfunction. Erection depends on an increased flow of blood that swells the vessels of the penis. Erectile dysfunction is commonly caused by narrowing of the arteries that supply the blood to the penis; it's associated with diabetes, smoking and high blood pressure. Sildenafil allows men to produce a sustained erection. This feat is accomplished by *vasodilation*—engorgement of blood in the penile vessels.

Until 1998, the only treatment for erectile dysfunction was painful injections (ouch) or awkward prosthetic devices (ouch). Sildenafil was first used in Britain as a drug to combat angina; it dilated the narrowed coronary arteries, allowing more blood through and relieving the symptoms. At that time it was found to have some unusual and enjoyable side effects, which led to its present use.

Sildenafil should not be used by people who are taking regular nitroglycerin by transdermal patch, paste or pills, because its blood-pressure effect is amplified by nitro. If you have stable coronary artery disease and are not taking long-acting nitro, but are using an occasional nitro pill or spray, then sildenafil is safe, but as a general rule it should not be used within twenty-four hours of nitroglycerin. If you use nitro occasionally, before taking sildenafil you should perform a screening test, such as running on a treadmill, to let your physician review your risk.

In studies comparing sildenafil to a placebo, there were an equal number of heart attacks in both groups, suggesting that when the drug is used in appropriate situations there is no significant increase in risk. Sildenafil may cause headache, flushing, stomach upset, nasal stuffiness and abnormalities of color vision.

10. Medications

Heart disease can be treated both invasively (with angioplasty and surgery) and non-invasively, through medication. Almost all patients with heart ailments, even those who have undergone an operation, benefit from drugs.

Most of us have a healthy fear of taking pills. Patients often admit to this distaste in embarrassment, with the mistaken notion that it's unusual. In reality, doctors are suspicious of patients who want pills. Respect for potential side effects is always warranted; medications should be prescribed only when the risk of not taking them exceeds the risk of taking them. For example, medications that lower blood pressure and cholesterol save lives. Although some people develop horrible and even life-threatening complications from these drugs, the overwhelming majority live longer because of them. Likewise, penicillin can kill people, but no one with pneumonia would refuse the prescription. No aspect of life is risk-free; the best we can do is choose the options with the lowest risk.

Blood Thinners

Why is it so important for heart patients to have "thinner" blood? Heart attacks are more than just a gradual, progressive narrowing of an artery. Blood flow is choked off abruptly when a cholesterol plaque in the wall of the artery suddenly ruptures. Plaque rupture triggers a cascade of events leading to the formation of a blood clot with the misguided intent of fixing what is broken. Spearheading this misadventure are platelets. They rush to the scene and organize the formation of the blood clots. Clotting works well when we cut ourselves shaving, but a blood clot in an artery spells doom. The clot occupies the width of the artery, cutting off the blood flow and causing the death of part of the heart muscle by starving it of nutrients. Irreversible heart cell death occurs within forty-five minutes. The longer the artery is blocked, the further the damage progresses outward, like ripples from a stone tossed into still waters.

The blood-thinner warfarin has already been discussed. In addition, there are other drugs in this category.

Acetylsalicylic Acid (ASA)

This extract of willow bark has been around for centuries, but it remains a powerful weapon against heart disease. Cheap, simple and effective, acetylsalicylic acid was isolated in Germany in 1892 and was synthesized in 1899 by a drug company. The first report of it being used for heart disease came in 1953, from Dr. Lawrence Craven in the *Mississippi Valley Medical Journal*, an obscure publication. He recounted his own experience with the drug in 1,465 healthy, sedentary men over a seven-year stretch. His finding was that not one single heart attack was reported. Although this unusual claim is unlikely to be totally true, the observation showed the potential effectiveness of ASA in heart disease. (In the United States, ASA is also called aspirin; in Canada, "Aspirin" is a brand of ASA.)

ASA has a wide array of biological effects. It reduces fever, relieves pain, is a potent anti-inflammatory and, most important for cardiac patients, thins the blood. By inhibiting platelet aggregation, it inhibits blood clot formation and reduces heart attacks.

Blood is composed of a liquid (serum) portion with numerous other constituents. Red blood cells carry oxygen. White blood cells fight infection. Platelets seal wounds, preventing blood loss, as part of an extraordinary and complicated blood clotting system. ASA inhibits the social life of platelets, preventing groups of them from congregating, so they can't clump together and prevent bleeding.

How effective is ASA at reducing heart attacks, strokes and cardiovascular death? Numerous trials involving many thousands of patients have shown its usefulness for primary and secondary prevention of heart disease. Primary prevention means that someone has never had the problem but is trying to prevent it. Secondary prevention refers to someone who has already had a heart attack, stroke, angina, angioplasty or bypass surgery and is attempting to prevent its recurrence.

For primary prevention, anyone over fifty who has never suffered a cardiovascular event but who has a cardiac risk factor (high blood pressure, diabetes, high cholesterol, cigarette use) should take one ASA tablet a day. The prescription for secondary prevention is the same: anyone with a history of heart attack, angina, angioplasty or bypass surgery should take a daily ASA tablet. Studies on secondary prevention suggest a magnitude of benefit varying from the prevention of fifteen events per thousand patients treated per year, to the prevention of forty events per thousand patients *per month*. Despite this wide variation, which is due to studies being conducted in different groups of patients, it's clear that ASA is very useful for heart attack prevention.

ASA is even helpful for someone in the throes of a heart attack; in that case the tablet should be chewed, to speed up the absorption of the drug from the stomach into the bloodstream. For someone having a heart attack, ASA is as effective as powerful, expensive intravenous clot busters like TNK-tPA and streptokinase. Its effect adds to the beneficial effects of these drugs.

The proper dosage of ASA depends on the indication for its use. For most cardiac problems, 80 mg a day is sufficient. Larger amounts—325 mg or 500 mg—provide no added benefit for platelet inhibition. However, for someone taking ASA for the first time, perhaps during a heart attack, a "loading dose" of 325 mg is advised, to achieve a rapid effect.

Although ASA is much more likely to prevent a heart attack than to cause serious bleeding, the fact that it can kill is undeniable. Although catastrophic bleeding in the brain (two per thousand) or stomach happens to only a few, it is difficult to predict which patient will develop complications. The higher the dose, the more likely it is that bleeding will occur. Using enteric-coated ASA reduces side effects. Fortunately, we now have other excellent drugs, with few side effects, that greatly reduce the risk of bleeding complications such as ulcers. ASA should never be used for children, as they can develop life-threatening complications.

Clopidogrel

Like ASA, clopidogrel is a blood thinner that inhibits the clumping of platelets, although by a different mechanism. Clopidogrel was a niche drug until the CURE trial, reported in March 2001, proved that when it was added to ASA it reduced death rates from heart attack, as well as further heart attacks. Previous studies had already shown that clopidogrel was as good as (if not marginally better than) ASA in treating heart patients. Unfortunately, clopidogrel is a lot more expensive than ASA, and its cost may delay its widespread use.

Beta-Blockers

Most heart patients are familiar with beta-blockers, a common and important class of cardiac medication.

Like all cells in the body, the cells of the heart (*myocytes*) have receptors for different chemicals. The receptors are akin to locks awaiting the right key. When the correct key is inserted into the receptor, it unlocks a cellular door, creating a chain reaction leading to a burst of activity within the cell. Cells have a host of receptors to fulfill a wide range of roles; a key may tell the cell to beat more strongly, for example, or to produce a certain chemical.

There are tens of thousands of *beta receptors* on every heart muscle cell. *Beta-agonists* are the natural chemicals ("keys") that insert into beta receptors. When a beta receptor is stimulated by a beta-agonist, it causes the heart to beat more forcefully and rapidly. When you are playing hockey, arguing with your spouse or anticipating a nocturnal tryst, beta-agonists are flying in all directions, inserting themselves into beta receptors. Any activity like this translates into a higher demand for oxygen. A steamship won't pick up speed unless more coal is shoveled into its furnace; the heart operates on the same principle. But higher oxygen demand creates problems for someone with coronary artery disease. Oxygen can only arrive via the bloodstream. If that stream is narrowed, demand outstrips supply, and the result is angina.

There are different ways of dealing with this situation. You can concentrate on chaste thoughts or sit in a room all day reading computer manuals, or you can take a beta-blocker, a drug that competes with beta-agonists. The heart now has two chemicals competing for the same receptor, with opposite effects. The beta-agonist carries the whip, flogging the heart to action; the beta-blocker carries a glass of warm milk and an old copy of *Reader's Digest*, soothing the heart into relaxation. When the beta-blocker occupies the receptor, it just sits there and occupies it, causing the receptor to "fall asleep."

Beta-blockers lower the heart rate and blood pressure, which in turn reduces the heart's oxygen requirements. They have been shown to reduce the chances of dying from a heart attack by 25 percent. Further, they reduce the odds of suffering another heart attack by about the same amount. For these reasons, they are a key component of drug therapy following a heart attack.

Beta-blockers are versatile drugs. In addition to being potent anti-angina pills, reducing the frequency and severity of angina attacks, they were one of the first classes of drugs proven to reduce complications from high blood pressure. Doctors may prescribe them for electrical abnormalities of the heart, such as tachycardias. They can also reduce non-cardiac problems such as tremors and migraines. Students have been known to take them before exams to alleviate anxiety. Performers may pop a pill before taking the stage.

Side Effects of Beta-Blockers

For a drug to have a positive effect, there is always the possibility of a negative effect. While more than 90 percent of people will feel better with beta-blockers than without them, some cannot tolerate the side effects, which may include impotence, bad dreams, depression and fatigue. It is difficult to predict who will or will not flourish with beta-blockers, but clearly some people should avoid them altogether. For example, asthma sufferers should never take beta-blockers as they inhibit the body's natural ability to widen narrowed airway passages; a number of deaths have occurred in asthmatic people who mistakenly took them. People with serious depression should also be careful, because these drugs can deepen the depths of their disorder.

Beta-Blockers in Heart Failure

The first reported use of a beta-blocker in congestive heart failure (CHF) was in 1973, by Dr. Finn Waagstein, in Sweden. He used the drug in a fifty-nine-year-old woman who was near death. She improved and lived until 1998. It has taken twenty-five years for proper studies, involving thousands of patients, to solidify the role of beta-blockers in managing CHF.

Beta-blockers are very useful in the management of congestive heart failure. However, because they reduce the strength of a heartbeat, their utility in CHF appears counterintuitive. In CHF, the heart is driven mercilessly by beta-agonists. By occupying the beta receptors, beta-blockers prevent the effects of the beta-agonists, and allow the heart to rest and improve. Within a month of use, the heart will beat more strongly.

Beta-blockers must be initiated very slowly in people with congestive heart failure. Close follow-up is necessary, because 10 percent of patients may develop worse heart failure. Despite overwhelming evidence of a reduction in mortality and the severity of heart failure, some physicians still find it illogical to use beta-blockers to treat CHF. Accordingly, only 50 percent of eligible patients are prescribed these drugs; a large number miss out on medication that could be life-saving.

Beta-blockers come in many shapes and sizes, but most end in the suffix *olol* (metoprolol, atenolol, nadolol, pindolol, practolol, acebutolol, bisoprolol, timolol). Some end in *alol* or *ilol* (labetalol, sotalol, carvedilol).

Nitroglycerin (NTG)

When not used as an explosive, nitroglycerin (NTG) is a very effective treatment for angina. It's an example of an older therapy that has remained useful under modern scrutiny.

NTG was first synthesized by an Italian named Ascania Sobrero in 1846, in his search for explosives. He experimented with the explosive called guncotton (nitric and sulfuric acids and cotton) by adding glycerin. The result was a combination of nitroglycerin and singed eyebrows. In 1867, Alfred Nobel built a factory to produce dynamite, a combination of liquid NTG and a type of mud. Nobel decided (a bit late) that he had done a bad thing, and established the Nobel Prize to balance his contribution to war with a contribution to peace. The prizes remain financed by his NTG profits.

In contrast to a homeopathic claim that because NTG causes headaches it should be used to cure them, the use of NTG in the treatment of angina is clearly proven. The first account of NTG use in angina was documented in 1879. In 1882 the Parke-Davis company began manufacturing pills, and it continues to do so today.

NTG widens the blood vessels. Which blood vessels are affected depends on the dose: low doses affect veins, and larger doses dilate arteries—most importantly, the coronary arteries. Dilation increases capacitance, allowing more blood to remain in the vessels, reducing the load on the heart muscle and allowing the weakened heart to rest. For this reason, NTG may be useful for conditions characterized by too much blood volume, such as congestive heart failure. Also, because dilation increases blood flow and oxygen supply to the heart, NTG can relieve the pain or discomfort associated with angina.

Nitroglycerin is quickly absorbed through skin and mucous membranes such as the inside lining of the mouth. It can be used in an ointment or patch applied to the skin, placed under the tongue, sprayed into the mouth or swallowed. In liquid form, it can be injected directly into a vein. The pill form contains a higher drug dosage than the spray, sublingual (under the tongue) tablet or skin patch, because when an NTG pill is absorbed from the intestine, the liver degrades much of the drug before it gets a chance to act.

Side Effects of Nitroglycerin

Nitroglycerin's main side effect, occurring in about 40 percent of patients, is headaches. In most cases they resolve within a few weeks. Approximately 10 percent of people cannot tolerate the constant pounding, and discontinue the drug. Another common side effect is dizziness, particularly just after standing up (postural lightheadedness). Palpitations may also occur. Some people develop a rash at the site where the patch or ointment was applied. Finally, there have been rare reports of explosion of a NTG patch near microwave sources.

During World War II, munitions workers who were exposed to NTG developed headaches on Mondays that resolved as the week progressed. This phenomenon was dubbed nitroglycerin tolerance. Constant exposure to NTG diminishes its efficacy; for the drug to properly work, patients must be free of exposure to it for ten to twelve hours each day. This "time off" is accomplished either by wearing a patch for only twelve to fourteen hours at a time, or by taking pills during only part of the day.

Nitroglycerin spray or sublingual tablets start to work thirty seconds to two minutes after use, peaking after about five minutes. If you try the spray or tablet three times successively and the drug doesn't control your angina symptoms, either the symptoms are not due to heart disease, or the "angina" may be a heart attack. Very rarely, someone with angina simply does not respond to NTG.

NTG should also be used preventively. Using a spray or tablet prior to starting an activity that predictably causes you angina (such as showering or golfing) may allow you to carry on without symptoms.

Calcium-Channel Blockers

Calcium-channel blockers are used to manage hypertension (high blood pressure), angina and some *tachyarrhythmias* (rapid heart rates). A cell is enclosed by a membrane that keeps all the cellular machinery safe, compartmentalizing it from the rest of the body. Embedded in the membrane are channels that function like doors, allowing ions and molecules to pass in and out of the cell. There are separate, specific channels for sodium, potassium, calcium and other molecules. If the wrong ion or molecule appears at the doorway, it doesn't get in. This allows the cell to regulate its own environment.

Arteries have muscle cells in their walls that allow them to either constrict or dilate. Calcium-channel blockers guard the channels of these muscle cells, barring calcium from entering. If the arterial muscle cells can't contract because they lack calcium, the arteries remain dilated, which lowers blood pressure, which in turn reduces angina.

There are two types of calcium-channel blockers. Some (amlodipine, felodipine and nifedipine) simply dilate blood vessels. Others (verapamil and diltiazem) slow the heart rate and dilate blood vessels to a lesser extent. Diltiazem and verapamil reduce the number of impulses that flow out of the heart's electrical generator (the sino-atrial node). In addition, they decrease the transmission of impulses through an important station in the heart's electrical system (the atrio-ventricular node), reducing the heart rate and resulting in less oxygen use and less demand on the heart.

Side Effects of Calcium-Channel Blockers
Calcium-channel blockers can mildly weaken heart function. This effect is insignificant if your heart function is normal, but if your heart is weakened from any cause, calcium-channel blockers can make it worse. Accordingly, someone with heart failure should use them with extreme caution, if at all.

Other side effects occur in 10 percent of people using calcium-channel blockers. Diltiazem and verapamil may lower heart rate and blood pressure too much, causing lightheadedness, fatigue and, rarely, collapse with loss of consciousness. However, the most common side effect is constipation, which can be easily combated with a few pitted prunes or a bowl of bran.

Amlodipine, felodipine and nifedipine can be potent treatments for high blood pressure, but they too may lower blood pressure excessively. In 10 percent of people, they cause swelling of the ankles and calves (peripheral edema) that can be severe enough to warrant stopping the medication. These drugs may also cause flushing, headaches and nausea. These three medications are not recommended as the sole therapy for angina, since they can, paradoxically, worsen it. When one of them is prescribed for angina, it is advisable to take a beta-blocker as well.

Angiotensin-Converting Enzyme Inhibitors (ACE Inhibitors)

ACE inhibitors are frequently prescribed. They can be recognized by their suffix *pril*, as in lisinopril, ramipril, captopril, etc. There are two major indications for their use: hypertension and congestive heart failure.

Enzymes are proteins involved in the manufacture of just about everything your body produces. They act as catalysts; if you wish to cross a deep stream but you can't swim, the enzyme might be the boat that transports you to the other side.

The angiotensin-converting enzyme (ACE) is involved in forming the compound angiotensin II, which raises blood pressure. (Angiotensin II was discovered simultaneously in the United States and Argentina in 1954. In the U.S. they called it renotensin and in Argentina it was named angiotonin. Put the names together and you get angiotensin.)

ACE inhibitors inhibit the formation of angiotensin II, resulting in lower blood pressure. As well, this class of drugs helps treat people with very weak heart muscles. Although ACE inhibitors do not directly strengthen the heart, they make it easier for the heart to do its job. If the heart is a fist punching a wall, these drugs change the wall from brick into balsa wood.

Up to 15 percent of people suffer from the ACE inhibitors' major side effect, a nagging, dry, persistent cough. Although annoying, the cough is not life-threatening. There may also be swelling of the mouth and face, which can be life-threatening, but fortunately this is a much rarer side effect.

Angiotensin Receptor Blockers (ARBs)

ARBs are used for high blood pressure and, to a lesser degree, for congestive heart failure. Like their relatives the ACE inhibitors, these pills inhibit angiotensin II. The difference is that instead of blocking its production, they block its action. Similar to the way beta-blockers block beta-receptors, ARBs fit into the receptor that angiotensin II usually occupies in order to act. This prevents the angiotensin II from increasing blood pressure.

This class of medications is relatively recent, and its benefits are trumpeted by the numerous drug companies that make them. There are at present five ARBs licensed for use in North America: losartan, valsartan, irbesartan, candesartan and telmisartan.

Drug companies profit from the research and development that went into the discovery and manufacture of their products through patent protection of new medications. After a certain number of years, however, this protection lapses. Then "generic" manufacturers are allowed to synthesize the drug cheaply and sell it at reduced prices. The original drug maker must also lower prices to compete, and thus has a much smaller profit margin. The patent protection on most of the ACE inhibitors either has expired or will do so shortly. Enter the ARBs.

Whether ARBs are superior in combating high blood pressure is unknown; however, drug companies profit by marketing them to widen their use. For the management of congestive heart failure they are clearly inferior to ACE inhibitors, but they do possess a superior side effect profile, with a negligible incidence of cough. While ARBs offer a slight benefit to a selective and small group of CHF patients, they are more expensive than ACE inhibitors and other anti-hypertensives.

ARBs should be used only when the alternatives don't work or cause too many side effects. However, as with all medical information, future studies may expand the clinical application of ARB.

Amiodarone

Amiodarone was first synthesized in 1967, in Belgium. Originally hyped to combat angina, it was not as effective as standard anti-angina medications such as nitroglycerin, beta-blockers and calcium-channel blockers. In the mid-1970s, however, amiodarone was recognized as an excellent drug to treat and prevent serious heart rhythm disturbances. Today it is known as the most effective drug for most atrial and ventricular arrhythmias, and is commonly used for a slew of rhythm disorders, including atrial fibrillation, ventricular tachycardia and others.

Amiodarone is a complex drug. Unlike most other pharmaceuticals, it dissolves in fat tissue. It therefore takes a long time to "load' into the body, especially in overweight people. For the first two to four weeks, high doses of up to one gram per day are prescribed to saturate the body fat. A typical maintenance dose is 200 mg per day, for five days each week. Unlike most drugs, which disappear from your system within days after you discontinue their use, amiodarone will remain in your body for months.

Side Effects of Amiodarone

Amiodarone has a number of potentially serious side effects, almost all of which are dose-dependent. The greater the cumulative dose over the years, the greater the risk of developing serious problems. This downside must be weighed against its role as an extremely effective anti-arrhythmic.

Side effects include altered activity of the thyroid gland—both too much activity (hyperthyroidism) and too little (hypothyroidism); liver disease (drug-induced hepatitis and even cirrhosis); lung disease (serious and irreversible pulmonary fibrosis); stomach upset; tremors that occur at rest, often in the hands, causing micrographia (small handwriting); photosensitivity (easy skin burning with minimal sun exposure); other skin rashes; and excessively low heart rates (bradycardia). Of these, the serious ones are infrequent, and were more common with the higher doses that were prescribed decades ago.

As with all drugs, you must assess whether the treatment (and its accompanying side effects) is better than the disease. In this case, the decision depends on the severity of the arrhythmia. The best philosophy is to use as small a dose as possible, and to ensure regular physician visits to identify any potential problems early.

Lipid-Lowering Agents

Statins

First isolated in 1976, HMG-CoA (3-hydroxy-3-methylglutaryl coenzyme A) reductase inhibitors are termed statins for colloquial use. Produced by fungi, these drugs interfere with cholesterol production in the liver. The liver functions like a factory; when it makes cholesterol, a series of steps must occur, and each is handled by an enzyme. By preventing one of those enzymes from working, statins cause a reduction in cholesterol.

Statins include lovastatin, simvastatin, pravastatin, fluvastatin, atorvastatin and rosuvastatin. Although each drug company likes to claim that its product is better than the rest, the differences are slight, and the most prescribed statin is probably the one marketed most effectively.

Statins' effect on cholesterol production depends on the dose; the higher the dose, the larger the effect. This is not proportionate but stepped—for each doubling of the dose, there is an approximate 7 percent lowering of LDL (the bad cholesterol). Studies show that statins can reduce LDL and total cholesterol by 25 to 50 percent, and that they are effective agents for primary and secondary prevention of heart disease.

Statins should be taken at night, before bed, since most of our cholesterol production occurs while we sleep.

Side Effects of Statins
Side effects are rare but may include a non-infectious hepatitis (liver inflammation) that will usually resolve when the drug is stopped. An even more uncommon complication is muscle inflammation (myositis), which causes muscle aches and a flu-like feeling. For a heart patient, the risk of a heart attack when not taking a statin is much greater than the risk of hepatitis or myositis.

Much ado has been made about an interaction between statins and grapefruit juice, discovered by chance in 1989. Grapefruit juice inhibits the enzyme CYP3A4 (not to be confused with the Star Wars robot) that breaks down many statins (lovastatin, simvastatin and atorvastatin) in the liver. In theory, this could allow the statin to accumulate in the liver and cause toxicity. Although there is a potential for interaction—it has been suggested that as little as 8 ounces (250 mL) of grapefruit juice can cause problems—the clinical effects of this interaction are by no means clear. Unless you drink bottles and bottles of grapefruit juice, or eat a whole bag of grapefruit, there is little cause for concern.

Niacin

Niacin is an effective lipid-lowering agent. More commonly known as vitamin B_6, niacin lowers LDL cholesterol. As good a medication as niacin is, it is very difficult to tolerate an effective dose, due to its severe side effect—marked flushing. Slowly increasing the dosage is one method of establishing tolerance to flushing, which does not usually persist as long as you continue the medication without missing doses. Taking an ASA tablet thirty minutes before a niacin dose is recommended. Within a few weeks, the ASA is no longer necessary. Niacin may be started at 100 mg three times a day, and increased gradually to 500 to 1000 mg three times per day. Although it is also sold in a "flush-free" preparation, niacin in this form is ineffective for lowering cholesterol.

Ezetimibe

Ezetimibe is a new type of cholesterol-lowering medication recently approved for use in North America. Ezetimibe inhibits the absorption of dietary cholesterol from the small intestine. This in turn reduces cholesterol delivery to the liver, and decreases the cholesterol levels in the blood. Ezetimibe has very few side effects, since it is minimally absorbed into the body.

Though statins are more effective than ezetimibe in lowering LDL cholesterol, the addition of ezetimibe is an excellent option for patients whose LDL cholesterol is persistently elevated despite taking a statin.

Jean was a seventy-nine-year-old widow living alone in a two-bedroom bungalow purchased with her husband fifty years earlier. Since her husband had died two years ago, Jean had barely been managing on her own. Her two daughters tried to help, but were too busy with their own lives to offer substantial assistance. For many years Jean had been suffering from chronic atrial fibrillation and hypertension, but her symptoms had never required hospitalization. Now that she was complaining of fatigue and palpitations, her family practitioner referred her to a cardiologist, and told her to take all her medications along, to show to her new doctor.

A taxi dropped Jean at the hospital entrance an hour before her appointment, and she sat in the waiting area clutching her plastic bag of pill bottles. When she was finally admitted to the doctor's office, she plunked the bag on his desk, and he looked up from her chart.

"I've been reading the notes sent by your GP," he began. "I understand you're having palpitations."

After a twenty-minute interview about her past health and present symptoms, and a short physical examination, the doctor opened Jean's plastic bag. Bottle after bottle rolled onto his desk. He collected them and carefully logged the name and dosage of each medication, and leaned back in his chair.

"Are you taking all these drugs?" he asked.

"I think so," Jean replied. "I might miss a few doses at times, but I get most of them in."

The doctor's tone was serious. "Do you realize how many different pills are here?"

"Not exactly, but it seems every time I go to my GP I come home with a new prescription."

The cardiologist looked at the long list he'd compiled, and read it aloud, shaking his head. "Some of these bottles are duplicates, Mrs. Robinson. I'm concerned you may be double-dosing a few medications. Including the vitamins, there are nineteen different pills in your collection. Are you planning on opening a pharmacy?"

Jean didn't laugh. She was too tired, too befuddled. Weren't the doctors supposed to take care of the prescriptions? She just followed their advice, or at least tried to.

The doctor took a practical approach. "I think we need to get someone to help you with these. I'm going to stop about half of them, anyway. You don't need them all, and no doubt some of your problems are related to side effects."

The cardiologist discontinued many of Jean's drugs. However, he wasn't confident that she would remember which pills to stop, so he placed the discarded bottles in a separate bag and offered to keep it in his office. He followed up with a polite letter to Jean's GP, explaining her situation and detailing the medications he stopped. Finally, he called one of Jean's daughters, and explained that her mother needed more scrupulous attention and care.

11. Complementary Cardiac Medicine

What is alternative medicine? The name implies non-traditional approaches to health. Some proponents of alternative medicine would have you believe that physicians, in their ivory towers, blindly refuse to acknowledge the health benefits of megadoses of herbs and vitamins, and non-medical practices such as trephining, cupping and rolfing. They claim that there is an alternative to seeing a medical doctor for your diseases and disorders; that you can cure yourself, without medical procedures or side effects, by following a simple and natural approach to wellness and disease. (This natural approach must usually be purchased from these proponents.)

The belief that one can attain optimum health by following the path of herbalism, naturopathy, aromas and other quackery has spawned a multi-billion-dollar industry of offerings. Like the cigarette industry, it generates profits at the expense of sound judgment. The proponents of these approaches may claim that physicians are driven by a need to control the health of others through drugs and surgery; that, fearful of losing their "market share," they subject their patients to unneeded tests and medications fraught with danger. To believe this, you would have to accept that doctors are misinformed about health and disease, are in a profession they know to be harmful and are driven by power and greed.

As scientific advances surge forward, they outstrip the ability of most of us to keep up. The pace of new discoveries can be intimidating. Alternative practices, on the other hand, cling to the notion that older practices are better and more natural treatment options. They constitute a rejection of scientifically based and usually (although not always) proven methods of treating disease. But trusting a practice because it has been around for five thousand years is illogical. Back then, the life span of a human may have been thirty years. Why try to recapture that? An intrinsically silly theory is a silly theory, regardless of how many people believe in it or how old it is.

The hallmark of alternative claims is that they are unproven; if the safety and effectiveness of a therapy are scientifically proven, the therapy is adopted by the medical profession, and it is alternative no longer. Yet proponents of these therapies resist randomized trials that would test their efficacy. They claim (conveniently) that the very nature of the natural treatment resists study. The consumer is left to rely on anecdotal evidence ("It worked for me!"), and may be persuaded to try "therapies" that are at best ineffective, and at worst harmful.

The distinction between traditional and non-traditional medical practice is artificial. As both camps would presumably agree, a therapy either works or it doesn't. A patient has a problem and wants it cured. The doctor offers a therapy. If the therapy cures the problem, it is not alternative. Even the most rigid alternative believers flock to the doctor at the first sign of real trouble. Few "natural healers" believe they can cure an actual disease. Most focus on chronic, non-specific symptoms like back pain, nausea and fatigue. If you have lower back pain and you rest in bed it will take seven days to resolve. If you see a chiropractor, however, the pain will be gone in a week! Cardiology is likewise awash with claims for dubious, potentially harmful alternatives. Perhaps the most popular is chelation.

Chelation

Chelation, advocates maintain, is more than an alternative to conventional cardiac treatment such as bypass and angioplasty. Chelation, they protest, is the *only* effective treatment for atherosclerosis, while global physician monopolies conspire to deny long-suffering cardiac patients this sole effective treatment. Fortunately, the chelation scam promises to abate soon, as studies continue to show no benefit from this dubious and potentially harmful practice.

Chelation uses a substance isolated in Germany almost seventy years ago, known as ethylenediaminetetraacetic acid (EDTA). EDTA binds certain ions in the blood that are then removed via the urine. Unfortunately, EDTA also binds many elements—including iron, calcium, magnesium, copper, zinc, manganese and others—that the body needs to function. Once they are attached to EDTA, these essential nutrients are excreted in the urine in huge amounts.

Chelation is an accepted and standard therapy for people suffering heavy-metal toxicity from mercury, cadmium and lead. But these are rare cases, specific to those who have worked with these metals in industries such as battery-making. Fortunately, workplace safety in North America has sufficiently improved in the past century to make heavy-metal poisoning uncommon.

Chelation proponents, who are lobbying for recognition from health insurance plans to sustain their practice, claim that EDTA transforms hard atherosclerotic narrowings into soft ones by stripping them of calcium. First, there is no evidence to support this theory. Second, even if it did work, it's the *soft* arterial narrowings that rupture and cause heart attacks. Making arteries softer is more dangerous, not less. But dead men tell no tales.

If a cardiologist wanted to make a literal and figurative killing, he or she would abandon hospital practice and open a chelation clinic. With the drawing power of a white lab coat and a cardiology degree, patients would flock to the clinic in hopes of an easy, painless cure for their damaged hearts. Since chelation therapy is not covered by health plans, the more treatments chelationists advise, the more you pay. The doctor's mortgage would be paid off by the end of the month, the kids would study in Switzerland and the garage would be filled with vintage automobiles. With hundreds of cardiologists across Canada, one has to question why none of them offers chelation.

The reason is that, unlike medications, angioplasty and bypass surgery, chelation therapy has never been proven to help patients with heart disease. People think it works, even swear by it, but health should rest on a more secure base than personal conviction and testimonials. If it were ever proven effective, chelation would be embraced. But the problem is not just that it has never been shown to be useful; it's that chelation may be harmful.

Tests versus testimonials

When you're living with fear and/or pain because of a health problem, it's tempting to believe a glowing recommendation from someone who claims to be a fellow sufferer. But personal testimonials are no foundation for health-care decisions. Diseases are complex and unpredictable, and symptoms may improve for many reasons—sometimes just because the person expects them to. All potential therapies must be properly tested before being offered to the public. Otherwise, treatments would depend more upon good marketing than good science. You may be willing to accept the "buyer beware" principle when it comes to buying a new washing machine, but your health requires consumer protection. Health is too important for us to allow charlatans to line their pockets while patients deny themselves effective treatment.

Yet numerous patients with documented heart disease are alive and well after embracing chelation. How do we reconcile this with the fact that chelation is unproven and potentially dangerous? As with all things medical and scientific, we must consider the statistics. What are the chances of living for twenty years with treatment option A versus treatment option B? Is there a difference in quality of life? (If a thousand people jumped from a three-story balcony and fifty lived to recount the experience, would you conclude that it was safe to jump?)

Modern medicine, like chelation and other dubious practices, must abide by the same principle. Bypass surgery has gone through countless revisions, over decades, to identify the most successful approach. Some practices have been abandoned after studies showed that they were useless or, even worse, harmful. An example is the Vineberg operation, in which the internal mammary artery was buried deep into the heart muscle instead of being stitched into a coronary artery. The hope was that the blood vessel would grow branches throughout the heart muscle, creating new vascular channels. But after studies proved that little or no clinical benefit was found, the procedure was abandoned.

Chelation needs to be studied properly under scientifically rigorous conditions. For example, subjects could be divided into two groups of equal number and composition. One group would be injected with sugar water, and the other group with the chelation elixir. No one in either group would be privy to which treatment they were receiving. After a set time—say a year—the groups would be restudied and the following questions asked: How many patients are alive in each group? How many are feeling well? If chelation performed better than sugar water, it would then be compared to more traditional therapies. If it proved no better, or worse than other therapies, it should be relegated to the medical dustbin, with the rest of the failed experiments.

The PATCH study, conducted in Calgary, Alberta, was reported in March 2001. It enrolled eighty-four stable patients with angina into a program of either chelation plus vitamins, or placebo plus vitamins. (Vitamins are a standard component of the chelation approach, possibly because most patients purchase them in the chelation clinic.) Thirty-three treatments were administered to each group. The study continued for six months, and showed no benefit whatsoever from chelation. In other words, people receiving chelation did no better than those given placebo injections. The PATCH study was small, but a good first step.

Chelation has no proven benefits, and great potential for harm. Besides encouraging people to delay proven therapy, the practice has been associated with low levels of calcium in the blood, kidney failure, low blood sugar, heart failure, liver failure and more. While clinging to a misplaced belief that chelation is cleaning out their arteries, patients suffer from progressing coronary artery disease, which increases their risk of heart attacks and death.

Garlic

Garlic is a perennial plant with extensive commercial cultivation in California. It's also often available in deodorized pill form on pharmacy shelves. Many consumers believe claims that garlic pills lower cholesterol, and dozens of trials have been conducted to look at this claim. Contrary to the conclusions of self-styled health experts—who stand to gain financially from their statements—no significant reduction in cholesterol has been noted after months of garlic use. This places garlic pills in the same bin of failure as many other herbal pseudo-remedies. The numerous Internet sites and health stores touting the cholesterol-lowering benefits of garlic are more than misleading; they are false. Garlic simply doesn't work.

Anti-oxidants

Anti-oxidants have been touted (by those who make them) as a cure-all for disease. In the world of unproven medicine, a pre-packaged pill, untested for quality control, can ward off tumors and disease like an ancient amulet. Is there any scientific truth to these fanciful claims? Can anti-oxidants keep us alive longer and maintain our health?

The term "anti-oxidant" is confusing, and doesn't conjure up a clear image. We must know what oxidation is, to understand the implications of anti-oxidants with regard to cardiac health.

The biochemical process known as oxidation must occur in order for living cells to produce energy (in the form of adenosine triphosphate, or ATP) from the food we eat. During this process, the food is broken down into smaller and more manageable particles, until ATP is made. ATP, the final form of cellular nutrition, keeps our engines running.

ATP generation is an oxygen-requiring (aerobic) process. ATP production produces harmful byproducts called reactive oxygen intermediates (ROIs)—also called free radicals, or oxidants, because they contain oxygen. ROIs are like the super balls that children love and adults hate; once they are thrown against the wall, the entire living room is a mess of broken lamps and fractured glass within minutes. In your body, ROIs "oxidize" important cellular components, causing damage to the cells' vital machinery. This causes injury and inflammation that may lead to tumors and arterial narrowing.

The body's natural defense mechanism against oxidants is aptly called anti-oxidants. Examples include beta-carotene, vitamin E and vitamin C (the body does not synthesize these three). Other anti-oxidants are glutathione, selenium, coenzyme Q_{10} and naturally occurring enzymes such as superoxide dismutase and glutathione reductase (which the body does synthesize). Anti-oxidants neutralize and destroy oxidants. So if oxidants cause disease, the theory goes, then supplemental anti-oxidants must prevent disease. If only life were so simple!

Vitamin C, Vitamin E, Beta-Carotene

A number of large trials have been conducted to determine the benefit (or perhaps risk) of supplemental anti-oxidants. Does the use of beta-carotene, vitamin E, vitamin C or selenium reduce the incidence of heart disease? Unfortunately, the results have been uniformly disappointing, but the question may still remain unanswered.

In the HOPE trial, nearly 10,000 cardiac patients were randomly given either 400 IU (international units) of vitamin E or a placebo pill daily. After almost five years of careful follow-up of these patients, there was no difference in the incidence of heart disease, stroke or cancer. Thus, it was reported that vitamin E supplementation appears to be useless in the management of heart disease.

In the Heart Protection Study, more than 20,000 people with various ailments (coronary artery disease, diabetes, peripheral vascular disease, high blood pressure) were randomized into two groups. Half of them received a daily cocktail of anti-oxidants (600 mg vitamin E, 250 mg vitamin C and 25 mg beta-carotene) and the other half received placebo capsules.

After years of follow-up, the results were a disappointment for vitamin manufacturers everywhere. This combination of anti-oxidants had no effect on heart disease or cancer. In fact, people on the anti-oxidants had a small but definite increase in bad cholesterol levels. Using the medications tested in these studies appears to be pointless. Sticking to proven therapy is the only regimen that a responsible doctor can advise.

The WAVE trial found that women had a greater chance of dying or suffering a heart attack when using vitamin C and vitamin E. A lobby group based in the United States, calling itself the Council for Responsible Nutrition, claims the results of this study have been exaggerated. The best advice, however, is to dispense with bottled nutrition, and focus on healthy foods.

Coenzyme Q$_{10}$

Coenzyme Q$_{10}$ (ubiquinone, or CoQ$_{10}$) is a popular and expensive product. Discovered in 1957, it is found in cellular organelles called mitochondria, where it is involved in energy production. People with congestive heart failure have low levels of CoQ$_{10}$. This deficiency can be improved with supplementation; however, recent randomized trials have failed to demonstrate any measurable benefit from CoQ$_{10}$ supplements in heart failure patients. Capsules of CoQ$_{10}$ have never been shown to improve heart function, or to alleviate symptoms, in those with heart disease.

The Future of Anti-oxidants

Until rigorous scientific testing proves otherwise, medical knowledge suggests that the best result one can hope for from anti-oxidants is expensive urine. Using anti-oxidants to ward off or cure heart disease is an irrational approach to health care, especially when we have proven, underused strategies to accomplish these goals, including exercise, diet and weight loss.

Although there are many books and Internet sites advertising the benefits of specific anti-oxidants, these resources are misleading, intentionally or otherwise. In the final analysis, doctors who recommend anti-oxidants for heart disease may be selling them.

Helen had spent most of her life battling her weight. Despite a bookshelf of diet advice, she stored an extra 30 pounds (14 kg) on her short frame. Helen's grandmother had died of a heart attack at age seventy-five. Helen's history of elevated cholesterol made her nervous, and now that her doctor had determined that she had high blood pressure, she worried about her own heart health.

"It's 162 over 92," her family doctor declared as she removed the cuff from Helen's arm. "This is the fourth elevated measurement in a row. I think it's time to treat this, Helen. Monitoring your blood pressure isn't useful as long as it remains untreated. Remember, you can't feel high blood pressure. But with every heartbeat your blood vessels are being damaged, increasing the risk of heart attacks and strokes."

Despite her growing fear of heart disease, Helen was reluctant to take medication for her hypertension. She hated the idea of using chemicals. Two years ago her doctor had recommended daily ASA, but she had declined the advice. At that time, her elevated cholesterol had been a concern. She had taken a brief stab at changing her diet, and had started an exercise routine, but her enthusiasm had waned after only a month. In the end, Helen had elected to monitor her cholesterol, rejecting the offer of medication. She felt the same way about her newly recognized hypertension

"I'd like to try to control it without pills," she informed the doctor.

The physician had heard this before. Helen had been her patient for ten years, and her records were full of Helen's blood pressure, cholesterol and weight; she was tired of cajoling deaf ears. It was frustrating to see her patient taking such risks with her health when options were available to help her.

"I don't think we'll schedule a follow-up, Helen. I don't feel I'm doing anything for you, and I have to be honest with you, this is very frustrating. If you want to discuss treatment options, give me a call, but otherwise, perhaps you should try to find someone else to monitor your condition."

Helen was mildly surprised, but she had her own plan in place. While she mistrusted pharmaceuticals, she had recently read a pamphlet touting the benefits of chelation therapy. A week earlier, she had written a $600 check for six courses of chelation.

The chelation doctor seemed full of care and concern; he was charming and persuasive, and talked with her for nearly an hour. He recommended twenty-five to thirty treatments, and assured her that her arteries would be cleaned out "just like new" after the miracle therapy. Before she left his office, he showed her an area full of vitamins and herbs, many of which he recommended to supplement his therapy. Another $220 later, Helen felt ready to face her risks.

Once the treatments were over, Helen felt better than ever. She was ready to continue the expensive chelation treatments. Unfortunately, her cholesterol and blood pressure remained elevated.

Three years later, Helen suffered a stroke. Paralyzed and unable to speak, she spent the remaining six years of her life in a chronic-care facility.

A Final Word

Heart disease is a widespread problem, and it is therefore crucial that we understand it. It is not only the aging population that is obsessively concerned about health. Heart disease is a great fear for all of us.

The first step to combating any illness lies in understanding its origin, how it progresses and what you can do to reduce your risks. Risk factor management is a cornerstone of treatment. Blood pressure control, smoking cessation, intelligent dietary choices, regular exercise and weight loss will dramatically lower your risk of a heart attack and its complications.

Health maintenance should involve consultation with your physician. Medicine does not have all of the answers, but advances continue to be made through scientifically designed, valid clinical trials to test treatments. Health may come in a bottle, but not an untested one. The results of proper studies will lead to an increase in longevity and improved quality of life.

Only forty years ago there was little to offer cardiac patients. Medical treatment has vaulted from advising six weeks of bed rest to curing heart disease with powerful new drugs and innovative surgeries. The next forty years will usher in dramatic new therapies with even greater benefit and less peril. Progress is inevitable.

Table of Drug Names

Generic name	Some brand names	Type
Beta-blockers		
acebutolol	Monitan†, Rhotral†, Sectral	
atenolol	Tenormin	
bisoprolol	Monocor†, Zabeta*	
labetalol	Normodyne*, Trandate	
metoprolol	Betaloc†, Lopresor, Toprol XL*	
nadolol	Corgard	
pindolol	Visken	
propranolol	Inderal LA†	
timolol	Blocadren*, Timolol†	
ACE inhibitors		
benazepril	Lotensin	
captopril	Capoten	
cilazapril	Inhibace*	
enalapril	Vasotec	
fosinopril	Monopril	
lisinopril	Prinivil, Zestril	
perindopril	Aceon*, Coversyl†	
quinapril	Accupril	
ramipril	Altace	
trandolapril	Mavik	
Calcium-channel blockers		
amlodipine	Norvasc	
diltiazem	Cardizem (SR or CD), Cartia XT*, Dilacor XR*, Taztia XT*, Tiazac	
felodipine	Plendil, Renedil†	
nifedipine	Adalat (PA, XL, CC), Procardia	
verapamil	Calan*, Chronovera, Covera HS*, Isoptin, Verelan PM*	
Diuretics		
amiloride	Midamor	
chlorthalidone	Chlorthalidone†, Hygroton*, Thalidone*	
hydrochlorothiazide (HCTZ)	Ezedrix*, Hydrochlorothiazide† Microzide*, Oretic*	
furosemide	Lasix	
spironolactone	Aldactone	
Lipid-lowering agents		
atorvastatin	Lipitor	statins
fluvastatin	Lescol, Lescol XL*	
lovastatin	Mevacor, Altocor*	
pravastatin	Pravachol	
simvastatin	Zocor	
bezafibrate	Bezalip†	other
cholestyramine	Questran, Prevalite*	
colestipol	Colestid	
ezetimibe	Zetia	
fenofibrate	Lipidil (micro or supra)†, Tricor*	
gemfibrozil	Lopid	
niacin/niacinamide	niacin/niacinamide†, Niaspan*	
Anti-arrhythimic agents		
amiodarone	Cordarone, Pacerone*	
digoxin	Lanoxicaps*, Lanoxin	
procainamide	Procanbid*, Pronestyl	
propafenone	Rythmol	
quinidine	Biquin Durules†, Quinidine*	
sotalol	Betapace*, Sorine*, Sotacor†	

Generic name	Some brand names	Type
Angiotensin receptor blockers		
candesartan	Atacand	
irbesartan	Avapro	
losartan	Cozaar	
telmisartan	Micardis	
valsartan	Diovan	
Anti-platelet agents		
acetylsalicylic acid (ASA)	Bayer Aspirin†	
clopidogrel	Plavix	
ticlopidine	Ticlid	
Nitroglycerin preparations		
(topical: nitropaste)	Minitran, Nitro-Dur	
(oral)	Dilatrate SR*, Imdur, Ismo*, Isordil, Monoket*, Sorbitrate*	
Anti-obesity drugs		
orlistat	Xenical	
sibutramine	Meridia	
Aids to sexual function		
sildenafil	Viagra	
vardenafil	Nuviva*, Levitra	

*Available in U.S. only
†Available in Canada only

Glossary

Angina: both a symptom and a diagnosis, angina is any symptom—commonly chest pressure, arm discomfort, neck pressure etc.—caused by insufficient blood flow through the arteries of the heart.

Angiogenesis: literally "new blood vessels"; a potentially promising therapy involving the creation of new blood vessels in the heart, by injecting genes responsible for creating blood vessels into the body.

Angiogram: a diagnostic test that allows visualization of narrowings within coronary arteries using X-ray dye.

Angioplasty: *See* **Percutaneous transluminal coronary angioplasty.**

Aortic valve: one of the four heart valves; blood crosses the aortic valve, and flows into the aorta and throughout the body.

Arrhythmia: a generic term for any rhythm disturbance of the heart, whether a skipped, rapid or slow heartbeat.

Artery: a blood vessel that carries oxygen- and nutrient-rich blood to the body.

Asystole: an absence of mechanical contraction and thus electrical activity from the heart, commonly referred to as a "flat line" on a rhythm monitor.

Atherosclerosis: a process in which the walls of blood vessels become full of cholesterol-rich matter, causing narrowing of the blood vessel and reduced blood flow.

Atrial fibrillation: a common rhythm disturbance characterized by an irregular and often rapid heart rate.

Atrial flutter: a rhythm disturbance characterized by rapid fluttering of the upper chambers of the heart. The heart rate may be rapid, slow or normal, and the rhythm regular or irregular. Atrial flutter is diagnosed on an electrocardiogram.

Atrio-ventricular (AV) node: specialized heart tissue that allows an electrical impulse to flow from the atrium to the ventricles, resulting in a heartbeat.

Atrium: one of two chambers of the heart (left and right) into which blood flows from either the head and body or the lungs. Blood flows from the atria into the ventricles.

Automatic implantable cardiac defibrillator (AICD): a device implanted in the heart cavity to sense abnormally fast and slow heartbeats. If the heart rate is too slow, it functions as a pacemaker; if too fast, it delivers an electrical charge to correct the abnormality.

Bioprosthetic: a biological substitute, typically from an animal. Bioprosthetic heart valves are often taken from cows or pigs.

Bradycardia: a slow heart rate, defined as fewer than sixty heartbeats a minute.

Bruit: the sound of blood flowing through a narrowed blood vessel. A bruit is heard with a stethoscope.

Cardiac: having to do with the heart.

Cardiomyopathy: a general term for a disease of the heart muscle that may cause severe impairment of heart function. Cardiomyopathy may be caused by any of a multitude of medical conditions.

Cardioversion: transforming a rapid and/or abnormal heart rhythm into a normal heart rhythm, electrically or with drugs.

Chelation: a treatment involving intravenous infusions of a substance known as EDTA. An unproven alternative or adjunct to the management of coronary artery disease.

Cholesterol: a type of fat, and a necessary part of all human cells. Excessive amounts of blood cholesterol contribute to artery narrowing.

Congestive heart failure (CHF): an inability of the heart to meet the needs of the body, resulting in inadequate forward blood flow and fluid in the lungs (pulmonary edema)—often, though not always, due to a weak heart muscle.

Coronary angiogram: a procedure that examines the coronary arteries under X-ray guidance. It involves inserting a catheter in the mouth of the artery and injecting it with dye. This detects narrowings of the blood vessel.

Coronary arteries: the arteries of the heart.

Coronary artery bypass grafting (CABG): a surgical procedure that uses other blood vessels to bypass a coronary artery narrowing, thus restoring blood flow to the heart muscle.

Coronary artery disease: narrowings (atherosclerosis) of the arteries of the heart.

Creatine kinase (CK): an enzyme present in heart, muscle and brain cells. Damage to any of these structures results in the release of CK into the blood, which can be detected by a laboratory test.

Diastolic blood pressure: the pressure in arteries when the heart is relaxed; the "bottom" blood pressure (i.e., the 80 of 120/80).

Dyspnea: difficulty breathing, shortness of breath (SOB).

Echocardiogram: an ultrasound test that examines the structural integrity of the heart.

Edema: swelling. Edema may be peripheral (legs) or pulmonary (lungs), or may occur anywhere else in the body.

Electrocardiogram (ECG): an electrical test that may diagnose various heart problems, including arrhythmias.

Endocarditis: an infection of a heart valve, almost always caused by a bacteria, resulting in damage to the valve.

Hematoma: a collection of blood, akin to a very large bruise.

High density lipoprotein (HDL): known as good cholesterol, HDL is a carrier system that transports cholesterol to the liver.

Hyperlipidemia: high blood fat levels.

Hypertension: high blood pressure.

Idiopathic: of unknown cause.

Ischemia: reduced (not absent) blood flow to part of the body.

Left atrium: a heart chamber that accepts blood from the lungs. Blood moves from the left atrium, across the mitral valve, into the left ventricle.

Left ventricle: the main pumping chamber of the heart. Blood flows from the left ventricle, across the aortic valve, into the aorta.

Lipid: fat.

Low density lipoprotein (LDL): known as bad cholesterol, LDL is a carrier system that transports cholesterol from the liver to the body.

Mitral valve: one of four heart valves; blood flows from the left atrium, across the mitral valve, into the left ventricle.

Myocardial infarction: a heart attack.

Palpitations: a subjective sensation of the heart beating. May be rapid, skipped, brief or prolonged.

Paroxysmal nocturnal dyspnea (PND): episodes of sudden shortness of breath that usually awaken the person at night. PND is a symptom of heart failure.

Percutaneous transluminal coronary angioplasty (PTCA): a therapeutic procedure that involves inserting a cylindrical balloon into a narrowed coronary artery and inflating the balloon to widen the area.

Perfusion imaging: a test that involves injecting the body with a radioactive tracer that is absorbed into the heart muscle, according to blood supply. If a part of the heart is supplied by a blocked or narrowed artery, this is detected on the X-ray pictures (perfusion images).

Platelets: blood components that clump together and plug holes in blood vessels, and allow blood clots to develop.

Pulmonary edema: a condition caused by fluid leaking from the blood vessels into lung tissue, resulting in shortness of breath.

Pulmonic valve: one of four heart valves; blood flows from the right atrium, across the pulmonary valve, into the right ventricle.

Re-stenosis: the narrowing of a coronary artery after a successful angioplasty and stent, usually within six months of the procedure.

Right atrium: a heart chamber that accepts blood from the body and head. Blood moves from the right atrium, across the tricuspid valve, into the right ventricle.

Right ventricle: one of two main pumping chambers of the heart, the right ventricle propels blood across the pulmonic valve into the lungs, where it receives oxygen.

Sino-atrial (SA) node: the heart's electrical generator; a collection of specialized cells in the atrium that initiates an electrical impulse that then spreads throughout the muscle, causing a heartbeat.

ST segment depression: an abnormality on an electrocardiogram; often a sign of coronary artery narrowing and, possibly, an indication of a heart attack.

ST segment elevation: an abnormality on an electrocardiogram; frequently a sign of a heart attack. ST segment elevation during a heart attack indicates the need for very specific treatment.

Stenosis: a narrowing, as in coronary artery stenosis or aortic valve stenosis.

Stent: a cylindrical steel mesh introduced into a coronary artery and deployed over a narrowing that has been treated with balloon angioplasty.

Stroke: a disease characterized by a lack of blood flow to a part of the brain.

Syncope: loss of consciousness.

Systolic blood pressure: the pressure in the arteries when the heart contracts; the "upper" number (i.e., the 120 of 120/80).

Tachycardia: a fast heart rate, defined as more than one hundred beats per minute.

Thrombolysis: a treatment for blood clots anywhere in the body. In a heart attack, thrombolysis may be used to dissolve a blood clot in the coronary artery.

Tricuspid valve: one of four heart valves; blood flows from the right atrium, across the tricuspid valve, to the right ventricle.

Triglycerides: a type of fat; high levels in blood are loosely associated with atherosclerosis.

Troponin: a component of heart muscle cells that is released into the blood when the heart is damaged, resulting in an extremely sensitive way to diagnose a heart attack.

Vein: a thin-walled blood vessel that returns blood from the head and body to the heart, after oxygen and nutrients have been removed.

Ventricle: one of two chambers of the heart that contract and propel blood into the body (left ventricle) and lungs (right ventricle).

Ventricular fibrillation: a serious rhythm disturbance that requires immediate treatment, without which death occurs. It commonly complicates heart attacks.

Ventricular tachycardia: a serious rapid rhythm disturbance that requires emergency treatment. It may complicate many heart conditions, including heart attacks and severe weakness of the heart muscle from any cause.

Further Reading

Colella, Tracy, Bernard S. Goldman and Suzette Turner. *So You're Having Heart Bypass Surgery; What Happens Next?* Toronto, ON: Script, 2002.

Myers, Dr. Rob. *Take It to Heart: Your Complete Guide to the Prevention and Treatment of Heart Disease.* Toronto, ON: ECW, 1998.

Ornish, Dr. Dean. *Dr. Dean Ornish's Program for Reversing Heart Disease.* New York, NY: Random House, 1990.

Sheps, Sheldon (ed.). *Mayo Clinic on High Blood Pressure.* Rochester, NY: Mayo Clinic, 1999.

Superko, Dr. H. Robert. *Before the Heart Attack: A Revolutionary Approach to Detecting, Preventing and Even Reversing Heart Disease.* Emmaus, PA: Rodale, 2003.

Index

For brand names of drugs, please see the table on pages 169–170.

flecainide 89, 102
fluid retention 114–116
folic acid 36
Framingham Table 26–28

garlic 162–163
gene therapy 68

headache, and hypertension 10
heart attack 6, 9, 61–65
  diagnosis 40, 63–65
  risk 25–28
  symptoms 62–63
  treatment 65–67
heart failure, self–management
  113–116. *See also* congestive
  heart failure
heart rate 87, 89, 148
heart rhythm 40
heart transplant 85–86, 125
heart, anatomy 1–4
heart-healthy diet 134–135
hematoma 76, 92
hemodynamic component 46
high blood pressure. *See* hypertension
high-density lipoprotein (HDL)
  23, 24
history, medical 58
HMG-CoA (3-hydroxy-3-
  methylglutaryl coenzyme A)
  reductase inhibitors. *See*
  statins
homocysteine, and heart disease
  35–36

hormone replacement therapy
  (HRT) 30–31
  and cholestrol 32
hot tubs 8
HRT. *See* hormone replacement
  therapy
hyperglycemia 29
hypertension 6–22, 57, 95, 149
  causes 13–14
  chronic 11
  damage from 11
  essential 9
  signs and symptions 9–10
  treatment 14–22, 147–149
  white–coat 11–12
hypotension 90

inflammation 56
irbesartan 150
ischemic heart disease 68
isolated systolic hypertension 10

kidney failure 6, 9, 11

labetalol 145
left anterior descending artery 3
left atrium 1
left ventricle 1
lipid 22. *See also* cholestrol
lipid-lowering agents 152–154
lipoproteins 23
lisinopril 149
liver 22
losartan 150
lovastatin 153

tachyarrhythmias 147–149
tachycardia 88
tai chi 19
target heart rate 47–48
telmisartan 150
thrombolysis 66
timolol 145
TNK–tPA 66
transplant 85–86, 125
tricuspid valve 2, 119–120
   regurgitation 125
triglycerides 24
troponin 65

United States, cardiologists in 66

valsartan 150
valve disease 119–132
   classification 121–122
valves 1–2, 13
   birth defects 126
   leaky 121
   narrow 121
   regurgitant 121
   replacement 129–130

stenotic 121
   surgery 129–130
valvular infection 128
valvuloplasty 124
veins 1, 55
ventricles 87
ventricular arrhythmia 151
ventricular fibrillation (VF) 104
ventricular tachycardia (VT)
   104–105
ventriculogram 75
verapamil 148
Viagra 137–138
vitamin C 164–165
vitamin E 164–165
vitamin K 98

wafarin 98, 100, 101, 124, 130,
   140
weight 16–18
   and blood pressure 17.
   See also obesity
women, and heart disease
   46, 165

yoga 19